Disaster Plann...g

MW00561854

Disaster Planning

A Practical Guide for Effective Health Outcomes

Mark Keim
Chief Executive Officer, DisasterDoc LLC; Adjunct Professor, Rollins School of Public Health, Emory University

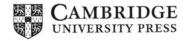

CAMBRIDGE
UNIVERSITY PRESS

University Printing House, Cambridge CB2 8BS, United Kingdom

One Liberty Plaza, 20th Floor, New York, NY 10006, USA

477 Williamstown Road, Port Melbourne, VIC 3207, Australia

314–321, 3rd Floor, Plot 3, Splendor Forum, Jasola District Centre, New Delhi – 110025, India

103 Penang Road, #05–06/07, Visioncrest Commercial, Singapore 238467

Cambridge University Press is part of the University of Cambridge.

It furthers the University's mission by disseminating knowledge in the pursuit of education, learning, and research at the highest international levels of excellence.

www.cambridge.org
Information on this title: www.cambridge.org/9781009004220
DOI: 10.1017/9781009004213

© Cambridge University Press 2022

This publication is in copyright. Subject to statutory exception and to the provisions of relevant collective licensing agreements, no reproduction of any part may take place without the written permission of Cambridge University Press.

First published 2022

Printed in the United Kingdom by TJ Books Limited, Padstow Cornwall

A catalogue record for this publication is available from the British Library.

Library of Congress Cataloging-in-Publication Data
Names: Keim, Mark, 1959– author.
Title: Disaster planning : a practical guide for effective health outcomes / Mark Keim, Chief Executive Officer, DisasterDoc LLC; Adjunct Professor, Rollins School of Public Health, Emory University.
Description: New York, NY : Cambridge University Press, 2021. | Includes bibliographical references and index.
Identifiers: LCCN 2021026973 (print) | LCCN 2021026974 (ebook) | ISBN 9781009004220 (hardback) | ISBN 9781009001960 (paperback) | ISBN 9781009004213 (epub)
Subjects: LCSH: Emergency management. | Risk assessment. | Disaster medicine.
Classification: LCC HV551.2 .K45 2021 (print) | LCC HV551.2 (ebook) | DDC 363.34/8–dc23
LC record available at https://lccn.loc.gov/2021026973
LC ebook record available at https://lccn.loc.gov/2021026974

ISBN 978-1-009-00196-0 Paperback
ISBN 978-1-009-00421-3 Cambridge Core
ISBN 978-1-009-00422-0 Mixed Media

Cambridge University Press has no responsibility for the persistence or accuracy of URLs for external or third-party internet websites referred t o in this publication and does not guarantee that any content on such websites is, or will remain, accurate or appropriate.

....

Every effort has been made in preparing this book to provide accurate and up-to-date information that is in accord with accepted standards and practice at the time of publication. Although case histories are drawn from actual cases, every effort has been made to disguise the identities of the individuals involved. Nevertheless, the authors, editors, and publishers can make no warranties that the information contained herein is totally free from error, not least because clinical standards are constantly changing through research and regulation. The authors, editors, and publishers therefore disclaim all liability for direct or consequential damages resulting from the use of material contained in this book. Readers are strongly advised to pay careful attention to information provided by the manufacturer of any drugs or equipment that they plan to use.

This book is dedicated to my best mentors, Kent Grey and Frederick (Skip) Burkle.

Thank you, Kent Grey.

Kent Grey was chief and organizer of CDC's first incident command center, the CDC Emergency Response Coordinating Group. As my first boss at CDC during the 1990s, Kent taught me the importance of objective-based planning – an approach that is still largely lacking among most disaster plans to date.

Thank you, (Uncle Skip) Burkle.

Skip Burkle was the founder and director of the Center of Excellence for Disaster Management and Humanitarian Assistance in Honolulu. As the thought leader in our field, Skip taught me the importance of measuring public health effectiveness – an approach that is still largely lacking among most disaster-related interventions to date.

This is for all the lonely people
Thinkin' that life has passed them by
Don't give up until you drink from the silver cup
Never take you down or never give you up
Never know until you try.
A song by America

Contents

Foreword

I thoroughly enjoyed reading this book. It provides a great, comprehensive review for many concepts that I've learned working in emergency and disaster management over three decades. It also covers the basic principles that I had learned informally along the way in a formal, modular set of lessons as well as including some critical principles that I had missed. Written by one of our nation's premier disaster response experts, the book progresses the reader through critical concepts, processes, and practices that make for effective disaster preparedness and response. Dr. Keim presents these critical concepts in concise, proper terms, and then shows how they work together. He builds on the basic, foundational principles, incorporating a very necessary, multidisciplinary approach. He also leads us to the next steps in our long journey of discovery for holistic, comprehensive disaster planning. These become like bricks in a wall held together with the mortar of a lifetime of experience, learning, and wisdom. To outline the important text would result in an entire book full of yellow pages.

A technologically complex, rapidly evolving community inherits fragility and unrecognized risk, and it needs more advanced, rapidly evolving approaches to disaster preparedness. In the years (almost three decades now) that I have known Dr. Keim, he has never been satisfied with the status quo. He has always looked to incorporate science with operations. We are fortunate that he was drawn to the public health and emergency management field, because, throughout his career, he has instilled the field with the structure of systems operations, systems architecture, systems engineering, rigor, and discipline. He moves us from the "portrait" paper form of plans to the "landscape" technological dashboards necessary for effective planning, preparedness, and response, and he adds a disaster planning warp drive for the journey. It is clearly not a simple effort, but it is what we need.

More than a guide, this is a plan outlining how our nation should capture its incident management planning and response "system." It is a roadmap into our future, combining the multitude of disciplines, processes, and best practices to secure the blessings of liberty through all-hazards disasters. It is a blueprint of how to build a comprehensive, extensible, agile preparedness and response architecture for all of our critical sectors.

Engage!

Dr. Duane Caneva

Preface

I first became interested in disasters at 3:16 p.m. on May 29, 1982.

That is the exact time when a killer tornado struck my small Midwestern US community – killing 12 people and rendering over 1,500 families homeless, including my own.

It was on that day, while standing there watching the tornado approach my home, that my survival depended upon knowledge that I had gained fifteen years before – what I had learned as a little boy reading a children's book about tornadoes. And even though our home was destroyed, my family remained safe and unharmed. To this day, I am compelled to share this story about how something as simple as a $1 children's book saved my own life and that of my family.

After experiencing this event in my early adulthood, I went on to a career as an emergency physician, disaster medicine specialist, and then a public health scientist at the Centers for Disease Control and Prevention (CDC) in Atlanta. While at CDC, I traveled all over the world studying disasters and the most effective means for managing public health emergencies.

During this time, I was shocked to find very little scientific information available about disaster planning. To this day, there remains very little empirical information regarding the effectiveness of disaster planning or regarding the quality of emergency operations in general. A few techniques are now widely used despite the absence of any measures of reproducibility of method or validity of outcome.

It is within this milieu of scientific uncertainty that I was asked to assist multiple nations in developing emergency operation plans – all in one summer! Thus, as this book will later describe, the planning system detailed here was born out of necessity. There was an immediate need to create hospital and public health plans for multiple nations and territories. This urgent need also presented an opportunity for in-depth study of the principles of planning and the application of these principles in real practice in over 200 subsequent examples all over the world.

After nearly two decades of facilitating and studying the practice of national level planning, I then had the opportunity to earn a graduate degree in business administration. It was the exciting capstone of theory that I needed to complete my practical experience. While studying at Emory University, I received the "Organization & Management Faculty Award" (an accomplishment that I can attribute to its close alignment with my own personal interest in emergency operations management and planning).

This book is intended to share with the reader the benefit of over twenty years of direct experience in real-world emergency operations planning. It is also intended to integrate this process of disaster planning within a larger context of business administration and systems-based theory for operations management, from which the modern science of planning originated.

The purpose of this book is to offer a somewhat disruptive approach to disaster planning. This "innovative" approach "boldly" proposes the use of century-old proven techniques for management of emergency operations. And while I note the novelty of this approach with tongue in cheek, it is also important to recognize that even a simple update in our current approach could easily result in measurable gains in the efficiency and effectiveness of emergency operations planning, especially as we move into the age of machine learning and automated planning.

Finally, this book was written during the world's largest disaster in a century ... the global COVID-19 pandemic of 2020. This entire book was written in a few months! It happened so fast that I felt almost compelled – driven by the opportunity to finally share *all* of this system, in one place, and in its entirety (as compared to previous intermittent publications of my findings along the way). Perhaps it was partly due to a myopic focus of pandemic-induced isolation and partly due to the decade of dedicated inquiry that had preceded the event. Now, after having percolated during my many years of study and practice, the entire draft manuscript simply bubbled to the surface like a spring that had finally been tapped. The rest I now defer to the thirst of the reader. My hope is to offer an oasis for those who may be called upon this journey or may have the responsibility of showing others the way.

Material Covered

The first half of this book includes an introduction to planning, along with an overview of the principles and practice of emergency operations planning. The second half of the book includes a detailed description of a standard process of emergency operations planning as well as methods for plan monitoring, evaluation, and improvement. The manuscript is also accompanied by a series of simple mnemonics, easy-to-read tables, and easy-to-understand graphics, all intended to facilitate practical usability of the book.

The content is designed to integrate disaster planning within the fundamental business principles of operations and process management. The ADEPT™ planning system is then described as a well-tested means for emergency operations planning that incorporates many of these basic principles within the context of group decision-making and multiagent incident command systems.

The book is composed of twenty-five chapters which are organized into five parts and two appendices. Parts I and II provide a basic orientation to the basic principles of emergency management and disaster planning. Parts III and IV provide a more detailed description of the ADEPT™ planning system, which includes the practice and process of plan writing. Finally, Part V describes the use of quality management systems for plan monitoring, evaluation, and improvement of disaster plans. The two appendices include an epilogue poem and a listing of over 300 definitions for key terms and phrases used in the book.

How to Use This Book

This book may be used both as a collegiate-level textbook and as an information source for professionals in the field. It is assumed that readers already know some of the basic concepts of emergency management. Prior knowledge of the scientific method and/or operations management would also be helpful but is not necessary.

The book is presented as a logical framework with a progression that first introduces the basic principles of disaster planning before describing their practical application. As such, one of the strengths of the book is that it describes many of the current practices of emergency management within a foundational context of operations management and empirical study. For this reason, even experienced emergency managers will likely learn new information when viewing the process from this perspective. In this sense, Parts I and

II are intended to offer a standard frame of reference for all readers, regardless of experience or perspective. They also offer a practical guide for plan writing and promoting a program of public health emergency preparedness. Parts III and IV are intended to provide step-by-step instructions for convening and facilitating group-based decision-making for risk assessment and emergency operation planning. Part V then describes a detailed system for plan monitoring evaluation and improvement in alignment with other modern systems for quality management (e.g., Six Sigma™).

A case study involving the fictional nation of Pyronesia is continued throughout the last half of the book. This ongoing case study allows the readers to consider the real-world application of these methods and techniques for risk assessment, plan-writing, implementation, monitoring and evaluation, and improvement as they are introduced in the book. Charts presented in the case study are realistic and based upon actual statistical calculations.

Appendix A is offered as an epilogue. This 100-year-old poem is intended as a final capstone to the book – intended to invoke thought and to serve as a poignant reminder of just how far we have yet to go with respect to prevention and control of disaster-related injuries.

Appendix B is a list of over 300 key definitions. One of the critical messages of the book is the need for standardization that will ensure reproducibility and validity of emergency operation planning. These several hundred standard definitions, drawn from multiple sources, have been curated and correlated to form a comprehensive nomenclature for the planning system. Readers are encouraged to pay special attention to these definitions, as they are mentioned and used in the text.

How to Use the Website Materials

In addition to materials in the book, there are also additional educational materials available via the Cambridge website: www.cambridge.org/keim

These materials include the following:

- A sample emergency operations plan: This example of an ADEPT™-style emergency operations plan uses Sphere Project standards as the subject matter content of an emergency operations plan. It illustrates how other standardized, hierarchical resources (e.g., Sphere Project) may be easily integrated as detailed disaster plan content.
- A complete training course for the book: These materials include a full set of 1,000+ PowerPoint slides for teaching the course, as well as a syllabus of learning objectives for the curriculum based upon Bloom's taxonomy.

This book provides access to an online version on Cambridge Core, which can be accessed via the code printed on the inside of the cover.

Acknowledgments

The author would like to acknowledge the contribution of the following individuals that made this book possible.

First and foremost, I wish to thank Alex Lovallo for his important and heartfelt contribution to this book's creation. Alex's work as a research assistant included literature searches, database management, and curriculum development. And he performed all this work under the duress of living in the Washington, DC area during the COVID-19 pandemic of 2020 and the Capitol riots of 2021.

Second, I would like to acknowledge the many individuals at the US Centers for Disease Prevention and Control that supported ADEPT-related training and interventions.

Lastly, I wish to acknowledge the many national partners that have participated in the implementation, evaluation, and communication of ADEPT™-related theory and practice. These include the nations of Palau, Micronesia, the Marshall Islands, China, Vietnam, Cambodia, Thailand, Laos, Uganda, Tanzania, Ethiopia, Democratic Republic of Congo, Kenya, and the US (particularly the Mariana Islands; Guam; American Samoa; New York, NY; Santa Catalina, CA; Virgin Islands; and Puerto Rico).

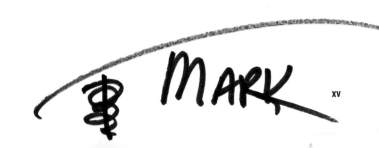

To Alex,
this book would not have been possible without you!

Thank you again for helping me share this with the world.

MARK

To Alex,
this book would not have been possible without you!

Thank you again for helping me share this with the world.

Mary

Chapter

What Is Planning?

1.1 Learning Objectives

Upon completion of the chapter, the reader can:

1. Define the following terms and phrases:
   - Accuracy
   - Activity
   - Analysis
   - Capability
   - Certainty
   - Contingency plan
   - Controlling
   - Data
   - Data schema
   - Deming's cycle
   - Effectiveness
   - Efficiency
   - Emergency operation
   - Empirical cycle
   - Goal
   - Hierarchy of hypotheses
   - Hierarchy of plans
   - Hypothesis
   - Incidence
   - Incident
   - Incident action plan
   - Input
   - Leading
   - Logical framework approach
   - Management
   - Management by objectives
   - Objective
   - Operations
   - Operations management
   - Operations plan
   - Organizing
   - Outcome
   - Output

- Plan
- Planning
- Process
- Productivity
- Quality
- Scientific method
- Staffing
- Stakeholder
- Strategic plan
- Strategy
- Systems theory
- Tactical plan
- Task
- Validity
- Work.

2. Compare and contrast the hierarchy of strategic, operational, and tactical plans.
3. Describe the management model known as "management by objectives."
4. Define the term "incident command system."
5. Recognize management by objectives as one of fourteen critical principles for the operation of an incident command system.
6. Describe the four steps of Deming's cycle.
7. Describe how the iteration of Deming's cycle is used to accomplish goals.

1.2 The Definition of Planning

Plans are designs for achieving goals.

Planning (the process of creating plans) is a fundamental property of intelligent behavior. All humans engage in planning. It involves the process of "deciding what to do and how to do it." The basic principle of planning is that individual and short-term decisions are coordinated to support strategic, long-term objectives. Plans provide the level of detail necessary for the accomplishment of a **goal**. The planning process usually begins with the most general concepts and leads to increasingly specific plans and tasks, resulting in integration between the parts.

Plans may be formal or informal. Informal plans tend to relate more abstract ideas and coalesce organically. Formal plans (i.e., those used for business and governmental purposes) are more likely to be documented and stored in a format accessible to multiple people across space and time. Plans provide a means for more predictable performance of plan execution.

1.3 The Hierarchy of Plans

Management universally recognizes three levels of organizational needs as follows: strategic, operational, and tactical [1, 2]. Each of the three levels is associated with a particular type of plan. This cascade represents a **hierarchy of plans**. The three hierarchical plans are interdependent, as they support the fulfillment of the three organizational needs.

Strategy is a plan of action or policy designed to achieve a significant overall aim. **Strategic plans** are descriptions of an organization's goals, the strategies necessary to accomplish those goals, and the performance management system used to monitor and evaluate progress. Strategic plans describe long-term goals and broad responsibilities for accomplishment. Simply stated, strategic plans tell us "why" (see also Table 24.1).

Processes consist of activities (i.e., tasks) that accomplish operational **objectives**. **Operations** consist of a group of processes implemented according to strategic objectives. Operational planning is a subset of strategic planning [3]. **Operations plans** describe processes, short-term ways of achieving objectives. Operational plans guide how a strategic plan is implemented during a given period. Simply stated; operational plans tell us "what" (see also Table 24.1).

Tactical plans describe directions (e.g., checklists, standard operating procedures, job action sheets), and short-term ways of managing resources (e.g., personnel, equipment). Tactical plans explain in detail how an operational plan is implemented during a given period. Tactical plans tell us "how."

On occasion, groups may also refer to the fourth type of plan, **contingency plans**. Contingency plans describe processes (i.e., short-term ways of achieving objectives) when our planning assumptions turn out to be wrong. Incorrect planning assumptions occur when unexpected events have disrupted a planned course of action, and alternate courses of action are required. Contingency plans guide how a strategic plan is implemented, given specific or unforeseen circumstances. Simply stated, contingency plans tell us "what if" when existing plans become inoperable or unsuitable.

Epidemiologists use the word **incidence** to describe the occurrence of an adverse event. Similarly, emergency managers refer to the term **incident** when describing an adverse event that necessitates emergency intervention. This intervention is implemented as an **emergency operation** managed using a standard **incident command system** (ICS). **Incident action plans** (IAPs) are plans that synchronize tactical operations and ensure support of incident objectives [4]. Emergency managers have developed a specific process and set of forms that assist incident personnel in completing the incident action planning process [4]. The approach to disaster planning offered in this book combines strategic, operational, and tactical levels of planning into one ADEPT™ planning system that may then be utilized at all levels, thus integrating international, national, state/provincial, and local plan stakeholders.

1.4 Planning As a Critical Function of Management

Plans are the foundation for the effective management of operations. Comprehensive plans often include strategic, operational, and tactical levels of detail.

Standardized operations are the key to reproducible quality in outcomes.

Planning should be deliberative and reproducible. Planning results in more efficient use of scarce resources than ad hoc allocations (thus its importance during resource-constrained emergency operations).

Planning is one of five critical functions of management (e.g., planning, **organizing**, **staffing**, **leading**, and **controlling**) [2]. Planning involves learning. Managers design systems in which individuals may work together efficiently. Managers also ensure that everyone understands the group's objectives and its methods for obtaining the selected aims. Planning involves decision-making, that is, choosing from alternative future courses of action. Managers compare plans with actual outcomes to guide corrective actions, as needed.

But before we take a deeper dive into the activities involved in planning, let us first consider planning within the context of management. In this book, we are considering a system for emergency management. However, these core principles for management (and planning) are just as applicable for *any* sector or management system (emergency or non-emergency).

1.5 The Definition of Management

Management is "the process of designing and maintaining an environment (or system) in which individuals working together in groups efficiently accomplish selected aims" [2]. Put simply, management is a system used to accomplish the goals of a group. Managers are responsible for the development, maintenance, and improvement of this system.

Industrialization occurred rapidly during the early twentieth century. Scientific advancements in systems theory began to impact the practice of management and professionalize the discipline. Frederick Taylor introduced a "scientific approach to management," which focused mainly on workers' tasks. Later, Henri Fayol (called "the father of operations management") introduced the process approach, which shifted from an emphasis on improving the worker's performance of tasks to develop management skills for producing successful outcomes [5]. According to Fayol, control of processes is the key to managing an operation's predictability and efficiency [2].

1.6 The Operational Approach to Management

Operations consist of a group of processes that are implemented by an organization according to a strategy. Since Fayol's work, this study of (public and private) business processes has developed into **operations management** [6]. In simple terms, operations management is concerned with designing and controlling the production of goods or services.

In this book, operations management includes designing and controlling services related to emergencies (i.e., emergency management), specifically health. However, this same planning approach is applicable for all emergency management and any public and private production of goods or services (including the emergent and non-emergent operations).

The fundamental approach to maintaining the quality of any set of operations begins with defining that set of tasks. Technically speaking, tasks are slightly different than activities. A task is defined as a piece of work to be undertaken or done. Work is defined as an activity that involves mental or physical effort to achieve a result. Activities are actions taken by a *group* to achieve their *aims*. In the United States, incident command systems often refer to these actions as "tasks" [7]. However, this book uses the term "activities" to represent the group's tasks.

In this book, tasks = activities

Systems are groups of processes that transform inputs (i.e., resources) into outputs and outcomes (i.e., objectives). A process is a set of activities that are interrelated or interact with one another. **Systems theory** is the interdisciplinary study of how processes transform **inputs** (i.e., resources) into **outputs** (products and services) and **outcomes** (i.e., **objectives**).

Operations management is responsible for this transformation. In the case of emergencies, managers use an incident command system to organize emergency operations. According to an organization's strategy, these operations transform human and material resources into services that address the population's acute needs. Incident command systems (ICS) are responsible for developing and implementing a daily incident action plan [4].

However, to be functional and reproducible, a process should be standardized, organized, repeatable, measurable, and aligned with strategy. These standards relate quality according to the following three measures: physical structure (i.e., equipment and facilities); process (i.e., how the system works); and outcome (i.e., the final product or results in terms of capability). In this case, a **capability** is defined as the ability to accomplish an intended strategic goal.

Table 1.1 depicts the relationship between processes, operations, strategy, and **quality** (e.g., performance).

Operations consist of a group of processes (i.e., tactics) implemented according to a strategy. Processes consist of activities (i.e., tasks) that accomplish objectives according to the group's goals. The performance quality for an activity is measured in **efficiency** (expressed as a rate of outputs produced per resource used). For objectives, measures of quality relate to the **effectiveness** of the operations in accomplishing the intended outcomes. Goals measure quality in terms of the functional ability to address a specific need or requirement of the strategy successfully.

1.7 Management by Objectives

Management by objectives (MBO) is a strategic management model invented by Peter Drucker [6]. According to the theory, being included in goal setting and action plans

Table 1.1. The organizational hierarchy of management processes, operations, and strategy

Level of hierarchy	Processes (i.e., tactics)	Operations	Strategy
Work organized by	Activities (i.e., tasks)	Objectives	Goals
Inputs	Resources	Activities	Objectives
Performance measures	Efficiency • Productivity • Cycle time • Satisfaction • Timeliness • Resource utilization • Cost • Safety	Effectiveness	Functional ability
Work resulting in	Outputs	Outcomes	Capabilities
Plan applicability	Incident action plan	Emergency operations plan	National response framework
Operational period	Hours to days	Days to months	Multi-year

encourage participation and commitment among stakeholders and align objectives across the organization. MBO, therefore, represented the first inclusion of employees as stakeholders in operational level planning. It also involves establishing a management information system to compare actual performance and accomplishments according to the defined objectives. Thus, MBO also helped to build systems for objective-based monitoring and evaluation of performance.

If you are involved in emergency management in the United States, you have undoubtedly already heard of the US National Incident Management System (NIMS) [7]. NIMS is an operational ICS that provides a standardized approach to the command, control, and coordination of emergency response in the United States. MBO is one of the fourteen fundamental principles underpinning the NIMS incident command system in the United States.

1.8 Deming's Cycle

But of course, MBO is not just about organizational structure. It is a system for decision-making. Figure 1.1 represents a simple two-stage process for defective decision-making. The **hypothesis** is an "educated guess" based upon subjective information. It is said to be "unscientific" because it is based upon a "hunch" and not measurable observation. Unfortunately, decision-makers use this approach to problem-solving all too often. It involves actions based on subjective information (e.g., a hypothesis), not data collection. Perhaps one reason this method persists is that it represents at least some small amount of planning before action! Many of us have worked with managers that subscribe to the erroneous principle of "Ready, fire, aim." It would falsely appear that at least having a hypothesis before acting would constitute an advancement in strategy. But it is a false choice, indeed. Actions (especially the life-critical decisions of emergency management) are best supported by evidence, not a hypothesis.

By the beginning of the twentieth century, managerial decisions involving the actions of increasingly larger firms were becoming increasingly more expensive and risk laden. Managers needed a better approach as they made decisions regarding how best to improve business operations. Figure 1.2 depicts DeGroot's **empirical cycle** depicting the **scientific method** as applied to decision-making. This scientific method (i.e., empirical method) forms the basis of all modern science.

During the early twentieth century, W. Edwards Deming began work on a scientific approach to modern management called Total Quality Management™ (TQM™). TQM™ represented the first of many subsequent models developed for process improvement (e.g., Kaizen™, Lean™, and Six Sigma™).

Deming's PDCA (plan–do–check–act) cycle is an iterative 4-step management method for the continuous improvement of processes and products [8, 9]. Figure 1.2 illustrates how **Deming's cycle** represents the scientific method applied to the management.

The concept of PDCA is based upon the empirical method of generating a hypothesis, creating an experiment, testing the hypothesis, and evaluating the results *before* committing to an action. In effect, Deming added the process of scientific investigation (represented as

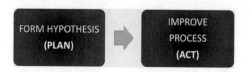

Figure 1.1 An example of unscientific decision-making

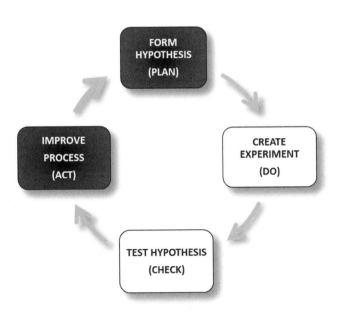

Figure 1.2 DeGroot's empirical cycle (with the Deming PDCA cycle inlayed in parentheses)

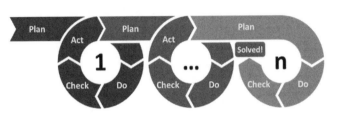

Figure 1.3 Multiple iterations of the PDCA cycle are repeated until the problem is solved
Source: Wikipedia
Permission: Open source

white boxes in Figure 1.2) to managerial decision-making. These added steps of scientific investigation typically include experimentation and hypothesis testing. These two additional steps allow managers to test their educated guesses before investing resources. This approach is beneficial in the case of emergencies when resources are characteristically constrained. The PDCA cycle is also useful for improving emergency response operations because it is intended to be repeated. This repetition creates a continuous quality improvement model over time, rather than a static current capability model.

Figure 1.3 depicts how the cycle is designated for repetition, adding the lessons learned from each iteration until the problem is solved or the approach is proven to be efficacious and therefore considered scalable.

1.9 Program Logic Models

An **analysis** is a process of breaking a complex system into smaller parts to understand it better. Program logic models are schematic diagrams representing the logic underlying the program's design, indicating how various components interact with the goods or services they produce and how they generate the desired results [10, 11]. Figure 1.4 depicts a generic logic model that can help clarify these assumptions for any public program. This figure compares the program logic model's six components to the three components of operations (i.e., resources, processes, and objectives).

Table 1.2. Example of a "log frame" associated with the Logical Framework Approach

	Description	Indicators	Means of verification	Assumptions
Goal				
Outcome				
Outputs				
Activities				

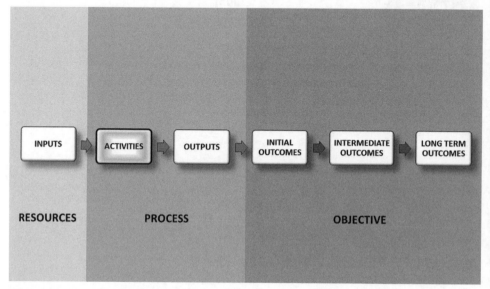

Figure 1.4 Example of a generic program logic model

Resources are inputs into a process by which activities create outputs and outcomes that meet the operational objective.

1.10 Logical Frameworks

The **logical framework approach** (LFA) [12] applies the program logic model to disaster assistance and development projects. It is also widely known as "objectives-oriented project planning." The LFA format (i.e., the logical framework or "logframe") is a 4 × 4 table consisting of project activities, outputs, outcome, and goals crossmatched to a description; indicators; means of verification; and risks/assumptions (shown in Table 1.2).

The LFA logframe provides a standardized format used to connect operational-level project plans to strategic-level donor goals for improved monitoring, evaluation, and reporting. The "logic" of the LFA works from the bottom up. Activities are accomplished to produce measurable outputs as a measure of efficiency. Outputs, in turn, generate the intended outcome as a measure of effectiveness. The accomplishment of all outcomes then results in meeting the strategic goal. This **hierarchy of hypotheses** allows for a cascading of measurable planning assumptions that integrate the informational needs of both strategic and operational-level management [2, 12].

1.11 Challenges of Effective Planning

"Effective planning allows people's needs, preferences, and values to be reflected in decision-making regarding the future" [13, p. 54]. "Planning is a social activity – that is, it involves people, and the results are affected by those involved and how they participate in the process. Good planning does more than simply identify the easiest solution to a particular problem. It can be an opportunity for learning, development, and consensus-building" [13, p. 54]. In essence, effective planning is reflective of effective management in that both processes relate to a system in which individuals working together in groups efficiently accomplish selected aims.

A planning process's outcome is significantly affected by how people are involved, interact, and communicate. Different people involved in the planning process may perceive a planning decision from many different perspectives. These participants are commonly called plan **stakeholders**. How stakeholders are involved is a critical factor in the effectiveness of the planning process [13]. This book refers to anyone involved in plan development, execution, or evaluation as a stakeholder of the Emergency Operations Plan (EOP). This book is primarily written for use by plan stakeholders to guide their participation in disaster planning (particularly for public health and medicine). Plan stakeholders may include public health and hospital officials, as well as their staff. In the setting of multi-sectoral planning, plan stakeholders typically include a much broader range of professions. Besides health professionals, participants involved in public health disaster planning should include a broad extent of capabilities. Following is a list of some of the most common stakeholders involved in planning for public health emergencies, besides public health:

- Chief executive's office (i.e., mayor, governor, president, premiere).
- Emergency management.
- Hospitals, laboratories, clinics, and home care services.
- Non-governmental organizations (NGO) and charities.
- Houses of worship and faith-based organizations (FBO).
- Public safety (police, fire, and emergency medical services).
- Public utilities: water, sewerage, power, telephone.
- Department of transportation, roads, and bridges.
- Department of education and schools.
- Public services: meals, social outreach, interventions.
- Military and national guard.
- Telecommunications, news, and weather agencies.
- Airport and seaport.
- Private industry and vendors.
- Community clubs and service organizations, community advocates.
- Traditional leaders of the community, community volunteers.

There are many challenges to effective planning. A few examples of these challenges are listed as follows [13]:

- Planning is often time-consuming and challenging to sustain.
- Many people have limited knowledge, experience, and time to develop, evaluate, or improve a plan's quality.
- Plans must often address a broad range of contingencies (tending toward a voluminous document) yet must also be user-friendly and easily accessible.

- Processes must be well-integrated and based on measurable performance.
- It is often tricky for planning committees to provide sufficient detail for many individuals' broad set of activities.

Existing models and guidance for planning have significant shortfalls [13]:

- Many plans tend to focus on content (or tasks) rather than the process (or management/coordination).
- Many plans lack clear indicators of performance and outcome or measures of effectiveness.
- Many plans are cumbersome. They tend to be large documents that are difficult to navigate.
- Some plans describe response strategies and fulfill legal regulations but do not address operational problems.
- Detailed operational-level plans are often not integrated into the overall strategies.
- Even where well-written plans may exist, the staff are often not trained regarding their specific roles and responsibilities according to the plan.
- Paper plans are bulky and difficult to distribute.
- "Disaster planning is an illusion unless it [14]:

  o is based on valid assumptions about human behavior,
  o incorporates an inter-organizational perspective,
  o is tied to resources, and
  o is known and accepted by the participants" (p. 35).

1.12 Four Characteristics of an Effective Plan

An effective plan has four characteristics: applicability, process, format, and content.

1.12.1 Applicability

Consideration should be given to the intended purpose of the plan, as well as its intended audience. Broad, strategic objectives are often most useful to top leadership and decision-makers, whereas managers and workers frequently use detailed tactical checklists and incident action plans. Operational plans tend to connect strategic directives with tactical details under one system of command.

1.12.2 Process

The process used is an essential determining factor of both the outcome of effective planning and the output of effective plans. It is through the planning process that we may manage (i.e., plan, organize, staff, direct, and control) the activities of planning to ensure outcomes with a high degree of **certainty** (i.e., **validity** and **accuracy**) and **productivity** (i.e., effectiveness and efficiency).

1.12.3 Format

The organizational format of the plan is critical for clarity of communication and ease of information sharing. Large amounts of information require a **data schema** to organize information for easy entry, storage, and retrieval upon command. This ease of access is critical during rapidly changing or emergent operations. Still, it is also just as crucial during the antecedent process of plan-writing when group review and negotiation of the plan requires simple, repetitive access to this information.

1.12.4 Content

Finally, effective plans require effective content written as strategies, objectives, activities, and responsibilities. The best creators of plan content are the individuals who are most often called upon to implement the plan's activities.

> Put simply, the best plans are written by the "people that actually *do* the work."

The most valid, accurate, and detailed content for activities to be performed in the plan originates from those same stakeholders responsible for implementing these same activities.

1.13 Questions for Discussion

Describe the logical framework approach in terms of:

- a hierarchy of hypotheses.
- integration of strategy, operations, and tactics.
- integration of leadership, managers, and staff.
- integration of disaster donors, response agencies, and victims.

What Is Disaster Planning?

2.1 Learning Objectives

Upon completion of the chapter, the reader can:

1. Define the following terms and phrases:
   - Catastrophe
   - Consequence
   - Core capabilities
   - Disaster (D)
   - Emergency
   - Emergency management
   - Emergency operations
   - Emergency operations plan (EOP)
   - Emergency operations center (EOC)
   - Emergency preparedness
   - Exposure (E)
   - Hazard (H)
   - Impact (I)
   - Mitigation
   - Natural hazard
   - Operational period
   - Population (P)
   - Preparedness
   - Prevention
   - Recovery
   - Response
   - Technological hazard
   - Threat.

2. Compare and contrast emergencies, disasters, and catastrophes.
3. Describe the five phases of the emergency management cycle.
4. List six functions of an emergency operations plan.
5. Describe the role of an incident management system for implementing an emergency operations plan.
6. List three examples of incident management systems used during disasters.
7. Recognize fifteen principles for effective emergency operations planning.

2.2 What Is a Disaster?

The definition of **disaster** now adopted by the United Nations [15] describes "A serious disruption of the functioning of a community or a society causing widespread human, material, economic or environmental losses which exceed the ability of the affected community or society to cope using its own resources" (p. 9). An event that does not exceed a society's capacities to cope is then classified as an **emergency** – a sudden and usually unforeseen event that calls for immediate measures to minimize its adverse consequences.

During disasters (in contrast to emergencies), organizations must [16]:

- Quickly relate to more and unfamiliar groups.
- Adjust to losing part of their autonomy and freedom of action.
- Apply different standards.
- Operate within closer than usual public and private sector interfaces.

Emergencies and disasters also tend to be conceptually differentiated from catastrophes. In a **catastrophe**, the disruption exceeds the ability of the affected community to cope, even using outside resources [17].

In a catastrophe (in contrast to disasters) [17]:

- It is not possible to terminate ongoing losses (even with outside assistance).
- Most, if not all, of the built environment, is heavily impacted.
- Local officials are unable to undertake their usual work roles, and this often extends into the recovery period.
- Most, if not all, of the everyday community functions are sharply and simultaneously interrupted.
- Finally, external assistance is not possible or is not effective in preventing excess damage and loss.

Emergencies, disasters, and catastrophes are thus part of a relative continuum of events that occur when a vulnerable **population** undergoes **exposure** to a "threatening event or potentially damaging phenomenon," referred to as a **hazard** [15]. **Threats** are hazards intentionally created by an adversary.

Hazards are commonly classified as **natural hazards** (associated with nature) and **technological hazards** (associated with human activity). Disaster **consequences** are the result or effect when a vulnerable asset (like a population, P) is exposed to a disaster hazard. The severity of these consequences is defined as a disaster **impact**.

2.3 Planning and the Emergency Management Cycle

The emergency management field originally described disasters in terms of a cycle comprised of four **mission areas** (i.e., phases) as follows: **preparedness**, **mitigation**, **response**, and **recovery** [1, 18]. Critics offer that this cyclical model may falsely imply the inevitability of disasters and that this classification may also infer a more distinct separation of the phases than the overlap which exists. However, categorizing these various emergency management actions into broad, time-based capabilities (e.g., phases) allows for more specific and focused planning to occur according to phase. As a result, disaster plans have, for the most part, been written for each one of these phases. However, this degree of specificity has also created some degree of confusion among the lay public and some responders as some tend to describe "preparedness plans," "disaster plans," and "response plans" interchangeably. Comprehensive disaster planning should include plans for all five phases of emergency management. Since this book pertains to the mission area of response, the plan is specifically referred to as an **emergency operations plan** (EOP) and is associated with a corresponding **preparedness plan for response** (PPR).

For example, recently, the United States has developed the following National Preparedness Goal: "A secure and resilient nation with the capabilities required across the whole community to prevent, protect against, mitigate, respond to, and recover from the threats and hazards that pose the greatest risk" [19]. This goal organized thirty-two **core capabilities** into five mission areas: **prevention**, **protection**, mitigation, response, and recovery [20].

As compared to the prior model that included four phases of emergency management (i.e., preparedness, mitigation, response, and recovery), this new national goal is designed to organize all core capabilities into five mission areas that ensure *preparedness for every phase* of modern emergency management (i.e., prevention, protection, mitigation, response, and recovery). Simply put, we must prepare to prevent ... prepare to protect ... prepare to mitigate ... prepare to respond and prepare to recover. Thus, preparedness is no longer considered one of the distinct phases of emergency management, but rather a cross-cutting goal for each mission area (e.g., each phase of emergency management).

2.4 The Preparedness Cycle

Figure 2.1 depicts the **preparedness cycle** as an example of the model used by many organizations to depict **emergency preparedness** as an iterative cycle [1, 4, 19, 21, 22].

It is also notable that these models are based upon a hybrid version combining the Deming cycle (Plan-Do-Check-Act) for quality control with Fayol's five functions of management. In the case of the preparedness cycle, Deming's "plan" stage is followed by a "Do" stage that includes sub-components (e.g., organize and equip; and train), which provide more tactical approaches to managing resources (e.g., staffing, training, equipment) in detail. These sub-components are notably similar to Fayol's five functions of management (e.g., planning, organizing, staffing, leading, and controlling). One may reasonably conclude that the preparedness cycle is Deming's quality control loop that applies Fayol's five functions of management to the goal of preparedness.

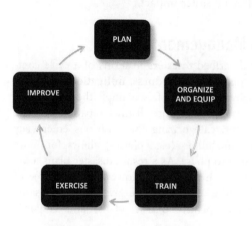

Figure 2.1 The preparedness cycle
Source: FEMA, 2010 [1]
Permission: Non-proprietary government publication

2.5 What Is Emergency Operations Planning?

2.5.1 Emergency Operations

In this book, our study of operations management focuses on designing and controlling the production of services related to **emergency operations**; those activities performed during the response phase of emergency management. However, these same principles of planning may just as easily be applied to the goals and objectives related to other phases (i.e., "mission areas") of emergency management (e.g., prevention, protection, mitigation, and recovery) as well.

2.5.2 Emergency Operations Plans

Emergency operations plans (EOPs) have been called the "centerpiece of comprehensive emergency management" [1, p. 29]. EOPs describe who will do what, as well as when, and with what resources, and by what authority – before, during, and immediately after an emergency [1]. According to the US Federal Emergency Management Agency, an EOP serves the following functions [1, 13]:

- Assigns responsibility to specific organizations and individuals for carrying out specific actions at projected times in any emergency that exceeds any agency's capacity.
- Sets forth lines of authority and organizational relationships and shows how actions are coordinated.
- Describes how people and property are protected in emergencies and disasters.
- Identifies personnel, equipment, facilities, supplies, and other resources available.
- Identifies steps to address specific mitigation concerns during response activities.
- Cites legal basis, acknowledges assumptions, and states objectives.
- Operations occur within a specific **operational period**.

EOPs are typically implemented through some formal or informal incident command system (ICS). Examples include the National Incident Management System (NIMS), the Hospital Emergency Incident Command System (HEICS), the Emergency Medical Services Incident Management System (EMS IMS), and the United Nations International Cluster Approach and Inter-Cluster Coordination System. This implementation usually occurs within the setting of an **emergency operations center** (EOC) or command headquarters (e.g., field offices and hospital command posts) where response-related data collection, analysis, communications, and decision-making typically occur. EOPs may be written at multiple public and private organizational levels, including international, national, regional, state, and local jurisdictions, and private institutions that may include entire systems or one installation. For example, the same ADEPT™ planning system described in this book has been used to develop EOPs as part of the US National Response Plan and district-level disaster planning in rural Uganda. This same process was used for planning a public health system for the world's largest mass gathering in China. Small individual hospitals have also used it in Micronesia [13, 23–28].

2.6 Principles for Effective Emergency Operations Planning

FEMA has proposed the following fourteen principles for developing an all-hazards plan for protecting lives, property, and the environment [1]:

1. Planning must be community-based, representing the whole population and its needs.
2. Planning must include participation from all stakeholders in the community.
3. Planning uses a logical and analytical problem-solving process to address the complexity and uncertainty inherent in potential hazards and threats.
4. Planning considers all hazards and threats.
5. Planning should be flexible enough to address both traditional and catastrophic incidents.
6. Plans must identify the mission and supporting goals (with desired results).
7. Planning depicts the anticipated environment for action.
8. Planning does not need to start from scratch.
9. Planning identifies tasks, allocates resources to accomplish those tasks, and establishes accountability.
10. Planning includes senior officials throughout the process to ensure both understanding and approval.
11. Time, uncertainty, risk, and experience influence planning.
12. Effective plans tell those with operational responsibilities what to do and how to do it, and they instruct those outside the jurisdiction in how to provide support and what to expect.
13. Planning is fundamentally a process to manage risk.
14. Planning is one of the critical components of the preparedness cycle (pp. 14–16).

2.7 Questions for Discussion

This book describes how a preparedness plan is developed for emergency operations in response to a disaster event. Compare and contrast how the content of the preparedness plan may differ for each of the five mission areas:

- Prevention.
- Protection.
- Mitigation.
- Response.
- Recovery.

Chapter

Planning As a Component of Preparedness

3.1 Learning Objectives

Upon completion of the chapter, the reader can:

1. Define the following terms and phrases:
   - ADEPT™ planning wheel
   - All-hazard approach
   - Capacity
   - Community preparedness
   - Disaster risk management
   - Disaster risk reduction
   - Early warning systems
   - Epidemiology
   - Evacuation
   - Integrated preparedness system
   - Mass care
   - Multisectoral approach
   - Preparedness plan
   - Program
   - Program management
   - Project management
   - Projects
   - Shelter in place
   - Sustainable development.
2. List seven objectives for preparedness related to public health emergencies.
3. List Lechat's four categories of preparedness measures.
4. Compare and contrast capacity and capability concerning emergency management.
5. List the "eleven 'E's" of emergency preparedness.
6. Describe the five mission areas of the US National Preparedness Goal.
7. Compare the old role of preparedness as only one of the four phases of the emergency management cycle in contrast to the new US National Preparedness Goal that applies preparedness to each of five mission areas.
8. Recognize how this preparedness goal concept differs in that it requires each mission area to create a preparedness plan and an operations plan.
9. List the five steps of the ADEPT™ planning wheel.

3.2 Emergency Preparedness

Although the terms "preparedness" and "planning" are sometimes used interchangeably, planning constitutes only one component of a comprehensive emergency preparedness program.

"Emergency preparedness programs are long-term development activities whose goals are to strengthen the overall **capacity** and capability of a country to manage all types of emergencies and bring about an orderly transition from relief through recovery and back to sustained development" [29, p. 253]. **Preparedness plans** are developed for each of the five mission areas of emergency management (i.e., prevention, protection, mitigation, response, and recovery).

Emergency preparedness programs should be one component of an overall **disaster risk management** strategy and should not be implemented as a solo project. A range of principles should guide emergency preparedness to protect communities, property, and the environment adequately. The approach must be as follows [1, 21]:

- Comprehensive.
- All hazard.
- Multisectoral.
- Community-based and user friendly.
- Culturally-sensitive and specific.

The **all-hazard approach** involves developing and implementing emergency management strategies for the full range of likely emergencies or disasters, including natural and technological hazards (e.g., conflict-related hazards of terrorism and warfare).

The **multi-sectoral approach** means that all organizations, including government, private, and community organizations, and traditional and informal leadership, should be involved in disaster preparedness. If this approach is not used, emergency management is likely to be fragmented and inefficient. The multi-sectoral approach links emergency management to sustainable development through the institutionalization of risk reduction and its principles in long-term development projects.

The concept of **community preparedness** is based upon the premise that the members, resources, organizations, and administrative structures of a community should form the foundation of any emergency preparedness program. As the saying goes, "All disasters are local," meaning all disaster responses begin at the local level [21].

3.3 Health-Related Objectives for Emergency Preparedness

Objectives of preparedness for health emergencies have been offered as follows [21, 30]:

- Prevent morbidity and mortality.
- Provide care for casualties.
- Manage adverse climatic and environmental conditions.
- Ensure restoration of normal health.
- Re-establish health services.
- Protect staff.
- Protect public health and medical assets.

In 1985, Lechat was the first to group preparedness actions into the following four categories [30]:

1. Preventive measures (e.g., building codes, floodplain management).
2. Protective measures (e.g., early warning systems, shelter in place, evacuation).
3. Response measures (e.g., rescue and relief).
4. Rehabilitation measures (e.g., shelter, resettlement, rebuilding).

Notably, the five mission areas of the twenty-first-century US National Preparedness Goal (i.e., prevention, protection, mitigation, response, and recovery) are now based upon Lechat's perspective of **disaster risk reduction**. As compared to the US's response-centric strategy from 1985 to 2015, Lechat's view represented what has also become the characteristic European perspective of disaster risk management, one that integrates pre-event prevention, protection, and mitigation efforts with post-event response and recovery.

3.4 Key Elements of Emergency Preparedness

Table 3.1 lists the "11 E's of emergency preparedness" – an easy way to summarize and recall many of the capabilities commonly involved in public health emergencies [17].

3.5 Case Study: The US National Preparedness System

3.5.1 Integrated Preparedness

The **integrated preparedness system** involves the coordinated management of preparedness programming for all five mission areas (i.e., phases) of emergency management (i.e., prevention, protection, mitigation, response, and recovery) [19].

Most disaster relief efforts are described as "projects" when, in fact, they are an ongoing **program** of work to realize a long-term benefit (i.e., a return to normality). Disaster relief programs also often include **projects** and elements of operational work.

Preparedness efforts must be implemented as integrated programs rather than a series of projects (i.e., temporary endeavors undertaken to create a unique result). Preparedness activities should reside within a program as a group of related projects managed in a coordinated way to obtain control not available from managing them individually. **Project management** focuses on the efficient creation of a defined

Table 3.1. The 11 E's of Emergency Preparedness

- Evaluation and monitoring of the hazard
- Early warning systems
- Evacuation
- Emergency operations planning
- Education and training
- Exercises and drills
- Engagement of the public
- Electronic media and communication
- **Epidemiology**
- Equipment and supplies
- Economic incentive

deliverable. **Program management** is intended to maximize the benefits realized with constrained resources in a changing environment.

3.5.2 The US National Preparedness System

As an example of national-level emergency preparedness systems, Figure 3.1 provides an overview of the US National Preparedness System (NPS), a standard process recommended for attaining thirty-two disaster-related core capabilities within each of the five mission areas that occur before, during, and after the disaster. According to this system, risk assessments guide actions that estimate, build, plan, validate, and update core capabilities. It is also notable that this model is based upon a modified version of the Deming PDCA (plan–do–check–act) cycle for quality control, where national preparedness capabilities are planned, performed, checked, and acted upon for each of the five mission areas (i.e., prevention, protection, mitigation, response, and recovery).

Notably, compared to the older view of emergency management as only four phases, the National Preparedness Goal recognizes the contribution of newer trends in disaster risk reduction associated with the mission areas of prevention and protection accomplished primarily before the disaster event. It no longer describes emergency management as a rigid cycle of preparing for the inevitable response and hopeful recovery. Instead, the goal is to prepare for all potential phases of an emergency, including those two new mission areas that may reduce disaster risk – preventing or protecting people from ever sustaining disaster-related losses in the first place. In effect, national preparedness aims to disrupt the cycle by preventing disaster-related impacts altogether.

Table 3.2 lists the thirty-two core capabilities of the US National Preparedness Goal (those eight capabilities most closely related to health outcomes are noted in italics).

Response capabilities represent the mutual goals shared by multiple sectors to carry out complex collaborative transactions during emergency operations. Table 3.2 provides one example of national-level, multi-sectoral core capabilities. These thirty-two capabilities of the US National Preparedness Goal represent the functional elements used by multiple sectors. Lead responsibility for accomplishing these capabilities is described according to a system of emergency support functions (ESFs) that provide a standard structure for

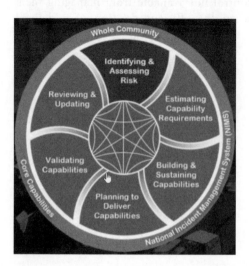

Figure 3.1 Six elements of the US National Preparedness System
Source: FEMA 2010 [1]
Permission: Non-proprietary government publication

Table 3.2. Thirty-two core capabilities of the US National Preparedness Goal

- *Public information and warning*
- *Health and social services*
- *Environmental response / Health and safety*
- *Fatality management services*
- ***Mass care** services*
- *Search and rescue operations*
- *Public health, healthcare, and emergency medical services*
- *Housing*
- Planning
- Operational coordination
- Forensics and attribution
- Intelligence and information sharing
- Interdiction and disruption
- Screening, search, and detection
- Access control and identity verification
- Cybersecurity
- Physical protective measures
- Risk management for protection programs and activities
- Supply chain integrity and security
- Community resilience
- Long-term vulnerability reduction
- Risk and disaster resilience assessment
- Threats and hazards identification
- Critical transportation
- Fire management and suppression
- Infrastructure systems
- Logistics and Supply chain management
- On-scene security, protection, and law enforcement
- Operational communications
- Situational assessment
- Economic recovery
- Natural and cultural resources

coordinating interagency support during an emergency incident [31]. ESFs are activated according to the consequences and needs caused by the incident. Many of these functions are cross-cutting, and it is common for multiple ESFs to be activated during a typical emergency response. Table 3.3 lists the fifteen ESFs identified in the US Federal Response Plan. Table 3.3 also illustrates how each of these ESFs may be further sub-divided into associated capabilities. These national-level capabilities offer a listing of capabilities to consider as disaster planners identify content for their plan.

"Planning to deliver capabilities" is a critical component of the US National Preparedness System and other national and international preparedness systems [1]. This book focuses on emergency response operations related to the core capability of ESF8 – "Public Health, Health, and Medical Services" as an example of this planning process. However, this same process is also applicable for planning any of the thirty-two core capabilities listed in Table 3.1. It is also just as applicable for planning related to all five mission areas (e.g., prevention, protection, mitigation, response, and recovery), not merely for emergency operations.

Table 3.3. Capabilities associated with emergency support functions of the US Federal Response Plan [31]

Emergency Support Function	Capability
ESF #1 – Transportation	Aviation/airspace management and control Transportation safety Restoration/recovery of transportation infrastructure Movement restrictions Damage and impact assessment
ESF #2 – Communications	Coordination with telecommunications and information technology industries Restoration and repair of telecommunications infrastructure Protection, restoration, and sustainment of national cyber and information technology resources Oversight of communication within the Federal incident management and response structures
ESF #3 – Public Works and Engineering	Infrastructure protection and emergency repair Infrastructure restoration Engineering services and construction management Emergency contracting support for lifesaving and life-sustaining services
ESF #4 – Firefighting	Coordination of Federal firefighting activities Support to wildland, rural, and urban firefighting operations
ESF #5 – Emergency Management	Coordination of incident management and response efforts Issuance of mission assignments Resource and human capital Incident action planning Financial management
ESF #6 – Mass Care, Emergency Assistance, Housing, and Human Services	Mass care (i.e., feeding and shelter) Emergency assistance Disaster housing Human services
ESF #7 – Logistics Management and Resource Support	Comprehensive, national incident logistics planning, management, and sustainment capability Resource support (facility space, office equipment and supplies, contracting services, etc.)
ESF #8 – Public Health and Medical Services	Public health services Medical services Mental health services Mass fatality management
ESF #9 – Search and Rescue	Lifesaving assistance Search and rescue operations
ESF #10 – Oil and Hazardous Materials Response	Oil and hazardous materials (chemical, biological, radiological, etc.) response Environmental short- and long-term cleanup

Table 3.3. (cont.)

Emergency Support Function	Capability
ESF #11 – Agriculture and Natural Resources	Nutrition assistance Animal and plant disease and pest response Food safety and security Natural and cultural resources and historic properties protection and restoration Safety and wellbeing of household pets
ESF #12 – Energy	Energy infrastructure assessment, repair, and restoration Energy industry utilities coordination Energy forecast
ESF #13 – Public Safety and Security	Facility and resource security Security planning and technical resource assistance Public safety and security support Support to access, traffic, and crowd control
ESF #14 – Long-Term Community Recovery	Social and economic community impact assessment Long-term community recovery assistance to States, local governments, and the private sector Analysis and review of mitigation program implementation
ESF #15 – External Affairs	Emergency public information and protective action guidance Media and community relations Congressional and international affairs Tribal and insular affairs

3.6 Planning to Deliver Capabilities

Until this point, this book's focus has been on the historical benchmarks associated with the development of planning and management systems and their application to emergency management. The focus is now on ADEPT™, an innovative system used for developing disaster plans that integrate emergency preparedness with mission areas of emergency management.

This system is represented as the **ADEPT™ planning wheel**. This allows the user to design and implement a capabilities-based plan for any of the five mission areas (e.g., prevention, protection, mitigation, response, and recovery) in a continuous quality assessment and improvement cycle. Note that the ADEPT™ planning wheel is, in fact, an iterative application of Deming's cycle introduced in Figure 1.1.

Figure 3.2 illustrates the five phases of the ADEPT™ planning wheel. This ADEPT™ planning wheel applies the following five phases:

1. Assess planning *assumptions*.
2. Create a mission area *plan*.
3. Check the plan for *gaps* related to planning assumptions.
4. Create a *preparedness* plan to correct the gaps.
5. Test the mission area plan for the *efficiency* of performance and *effectiveness* of outcomes.

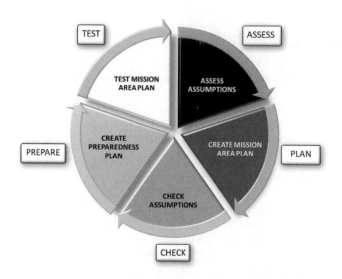

Figure 3.2 The ADEPT™ planning wheel

The ADEPT™ planning wheel is discussed in detail in Chapter 16, but suffice it to say for now that disaster planning begins with an assessment of the planning assumptions (e.g., risk assessment, functional analysis, and capacity inventory). Using these planning assumptions to represent the "one single truth," stakeholders then create a plan for one of the five mission areas (e.g., an emergency operations plan – EOP). Once drafted, the resultant plan is then checked for gaps compared to the expected needs and resources estimated in the planning assumptions. This gap analysis is then used to guide creating a preparedness plan that fills those gaps. Finally, both plans' effectiveness and efficiency are tested using simulations, exercises, or real events as part of a more comprehensive multi-year preparedness program.

This approach offers practitioners a simple roadmap for building and improving disaster preparedness programs. This process should be repeated, at minimum, on an annual basis. High-profile or rapidly changing events (such as large mass gatherings or high-threat environments) may require a more frequent repetitive cycle.

This model also aligns the US National Preparedness System with Deming's cycle for quality control during operations. Thus, the ADEPT™ planning wheel integrates operational-level control theory with evidence-based national-level preparedness strategies.

3.7 Questions for Discussion

- Compare and contrast Lechat's four categories of preparedness measures to the five mission areas of the US National Preparedness Goal.
- Compare and contrast project management with program management in terms of budget, scope, and timeframe.
- Describe the divergence of US and European models for preparedness after 1985 and then their reconvergence in 2015. Why do you think they diverged? Why did they reconverge?

4 A Capability-Based Approach for Emergency Preparedness

4.1 Learning Objectives

Upon completion of the chapter, the reader can:

1. Define the following terms and phrases:
   - Absorptive capacity
   - Adaptive capacity
   - Evaluation
   - Monitoring
   - Monitoring and evaluation (M&E)
   - Operational debriefing
   - Resilience
   - Systems analysis
   - Transformative capacity.
2. Recognize the public health consequences of disasters caused by natural and technological hazards.
3. Describe how the public health consequences are the same for most disasters and differ mostly in scale.
4. Recognize capabilities that address the public health consequences of disasters.
5. Compare and contrast the terms "capability" and "capacity" in terms of disaster planning.
6. Describe the use of hazard–impact matrices to prioritize disaster hazards.
7. Describe how a gap analysis compares current capacities to predicted capacities.
8. Describe absorptive, adaptive, and transformative capacity and give examples of each.
9. List twelve elements of an emergency preparedness program.
10. Compare and contrast monitoring and evaluation.

4.2 The Public Health Consequences of Disasters

Populations at risk for disasters may face many vastly different hazards and threats within a nearly infinite set of unpredictable scenarios [21]. This unpredictability is poorly suited to scenario-based approaches for emergency management (i.e., approaches focused on specific prioritized hazards) [32]. While the hazards that cause disasters may vary considerably, fortunately the potential public health consequences and subsequent public health and medical needs of the population do not [1, 21, 33]. For example, warfare, chemical releases, floods, hurricanes, and earthquakes all displace people from their homes. These various disaster hazards require the same public health capability of shelter, with only minor adjustments for the impact (severity according to hazard rapidity of onset, scale, duration, location, and intensity). Regardless of the hazard, functional analyses have revealed that these disasters cause fifteen public health consequences addressed by thirty-two categories of public health and medical capabilities [21]. Tables 4.1 and 4.2 list the public health consequences most commonly associated with significant natural and technological disasters, respectively [17, 21]. Note that for most of the disaster hazards represented in these tables, variation exists only for the relative degree of impact for each of the public health consequences. Thus, the all-hazard preparedness program focuses not on the specific hazard but rather on addressing each of the expected public health and medical consequences. These consequences are managed through a projection of an inventory of emergency response capabilities.

Table 4.3 lists the public health capabilities necessary to address those public health consequences listed in Tables 4.1 and 4.2 that are most commonly addressed in disaster response [21]. Thus, an effective emergency response can be developed by implementing a preparedness program that builds capacity for each of the capabilities listed in Table 4.3 (in most cases, regardless of the hazard). An effective public health and medical preparedness program applies the six elements of the US National Preparedness System (listed in Figure 3.1) according to the five steps of the preparedness cycle (listed in Figure 2.1) toward the goal of building capacity for each of the capabilities listed in Table 4.3 [21].

4.3 Comparing Capability and Capacity

Using an all-hazard approach, societies and organizations apply deliberate planning to prepare for and respond to disasters by applying their inherent capabilities to all disaster risks, regardless of priority. A capability is defined as the "ability to achieve a desired operational effect under specified standards and conditions through combinations of means and ways to perform a set of tasks" [32, p. 12]. The capability-based approach to planning was initially proposed by Nobel Prize-winning economists Sen and Nussbaum [36]. Murphy and Gardoni also proposed using a capability-based approach to measure hazard impact and direct risk analysis and hazard mitigation efforts [61, 62]. Defense agencies have extensively applied capability-based approaches to risk management to address the challenges of uncertainty related to hazards involving asymmetrical warfare (i.e., terrorism) [54, 55].

Like preparedness, capacity is a cross-cutting asset applied throughout all five mission areas of emergency management, not merely response.

Capacity is the (rate at which) the "combination of all the strengths, attributes, and resources available within a community, society or organization can be used to achieve agreed goals" [15, pp. 5–6]. Although the two terms may be erroneously used interchangeably, it is crucial to differentiate capability from capacity. While capability is the *ability* to achieve the desired goal, capacity is the upper limit of all the strengths, attributes, and resources available to achieve that goal [15]. Capacity is a rate that measures the performance of a capability over time. Let us consider drinking water as an example. Water has the "capability" to hydrate our body – a measurable *outcome*. But one liter of water is not of sufficient capacity to hydrate our body for an entire day. That would require a capacity of five liters per person per day (a measurable *output*). Populations apply capacity to reduce the risk of adverse outcomes before, during, and after the disaster event itself.

Table 4.1. The relative public health impact of select natural disaster hazards

Public Health Consequence	Infectious	Environmental					
	Epidemics	Flood	Heat wave	Storm	Tropical Cyclone	Drought	Wildfire
Number of deaths	Can be many	Few, but many in poor nations	Can be many (especially in large urban areas)	Few	Few, but many in poor nations	Few, but many in poor nations	Few
Severe injuries	Insignificant	Few	Can be many (heat illness)	Few	Few	Unlikely	Few
Loss of clean water	Insignificant	Focal to widespread	Insignificant	Focal	Focal to widespread	Widespread	Focal
Loss of shelter	Insignificant	Focal to widespread	Insignificant	Focal	Focal to widespread	Focal to widespread	Focal
Loss of personal/household goods	Insignificant	Focal to widespread	Insignificant	Focal	Focal to widespread	Focal to widespread	Focal
Major population movements	Insignificant	Focal to widespread	Insignificant	Focal	Focal to widespread	Focal to widespread	Focal
Loss of routine hygiene	Insignificant	Focal to widespread	Insignificant	Focal	Focal to widespread	Widespread	Focal
Loss of sanitation	Insignificant	Focal to widespread	Insignificant	Focal	Focal to widespread	Focal	Focal
Disruption of solid waste management	Insignificant	Focal to widespread	Insignificant	Focal	Focal to widespread	Focal	Focal
Public concern for safety	Moderate	Moderate to high	Low to moderate	Low to moderate	High	Low to moderate	Moderate to High

Table 4.1. (cont.)

Public Health Consequence	Infectious	Environmental					
	Epidemics	Flood	Heat wave	Storm	Tropical Cyclone	Drought	Wildfire
Increased pests	Insignificant	Focal to widespread	Insignificant	Focal	Focal to widespread	Focal to widespread	Unlikely
Loss or damage of health care system	Insignificant	Focal to widespread	Insignificant	Focal	Focal to widespread	Focal	Focal to widespread
Worsening of chronic illnesses	Focal to widespread	Focal to widespread	Focal to widespread	Focal	Focal to widespread	Widespread	Focal to widespread
Loss of electrical power	Insignificant	Focal to widespread	Occasionally focal	Focal	Focal to widespread	Focal	Unlikely
Toxic exposures	Insignificant	Widespread for CO poisoning	Insignificant	Focal for CO poisoning	Widespread for CO poisoning	Focal	Widespread for air
Food scarcity	Insignificant	Focal to widespread	Insignificant	Insignificant	Common in low-lying coastal areas	Widespread in poor nations	Focal

Source: With permission from Elsevier

Table 4.2. The relative public health impact of select technological disaster hazards

Public Health Consequence	Terrorism/Conflict				
	Industrial				
	Toxicological	Thermal	Mechanical		
	Hazardous material release	Urban fire	Explosions/ bombings	Transport crash	Structural failure
Deaths	Moderate to many	Few to moderate	Moderate to many	Few to moderate	Moderate to many
Severe injuries	Moderate to many	Moderate to many	Moderate to many	Moderate to many	Moderate to many
Loss of clean water	Focal	Focal	Focal	Focal	Focal
Loss of shelter	Focal	Focal	Focal	Focal	Focal
Loss of personal and household goods	Focal	Focal	Focal	Focal	Focal
Major population movements	Focal	Focal	Focal	Focal	Focal
Loss of routine hygiene	Focal	Focal	Focal	Focal	Focal
Loss of sanitation	Focal	Focal	Focal	Focal	Focal
Disruption of solid waste management	Unlikely	Unlikely	Unlikely	Unlikely	Unlikely
Public concern for safety	High	High	High	High	High
Increased pests and vectors	Unlikely	Unlikely	Unlikely	Unlikely	Unlikely
Loss of and/or damage to health care system	Focal	Focal	Focal	Focal	Focal
Worsening of existing chronic illnesses	Focal to widespread	Focal to widespread	Focal	Focal	Focal
Loss of electricity	Focal	Focal	Focal	Focal	Focal
Toxic exposures	Focal to widespread	Focal to widespread	Focal	Focal	Focal
Food scarcity	Unlikely	Unlikely	Unlikely	Unlikely	Unlikely

Source: Permission granted by Elsevier

Table 4.3. Public health consequences and capabilities associated with all disasters

Public health consequences	Core capabilities affecting public health
Surge of administrative, informational, and operational needs	Resource management Information sharing § Emergency operations coordination § Responder safety and health § Occupational health and safety Business continuity Volunteer management § Situational awareness
Deaths	Fatality management § / Mortuary care Social services Mental health services
Illness and injuries	Health services Mental health services Injury prevention and control Public health surveillance § / Epidemiological investigation Disease prevention and control Medical countermeasure dispensing § Medical material management and distribution § Public health laboratory testing § Medical surge § Non-pharmaceutical interventions (isolation, quarantine, social distancing, travel restriction/advice) §
Loss of clean water	Water, sanitation, and hygiene (WASH) Health services (e.g., hospitals, dialysis units)
Loss of shelter	Mass care § / Shelter and settlement Social services Security
Loss of personal and household goods	Replacement of personal and household goods
Loss of sanitation and routine hygiene	Sanitation, excreta disposal, and hygiene promotion Non-pharmaceutical interventions (hygiène) §
Disruption of solid waste management	Solid waste management
Public concern for safety	Risk communication / Emergency public information and warning § Security
Increased pests and vectors	Pest and vector control
Loss or damage of health care system	Health system and infrastructure support Reproductive health services Health services
Worsening of chronic illnesses	Health services

Table 4.3. (cont.)

Public health consequences	Core capabilities affecting public health
Food scarcity	Food safety, food security, and nutrition
Standing surface water	Public works and engineering
Toxic exposures	Risk assessment and exposure modeling
	Population protection measures (evacuation/shelter in place)
	Health services
	Hazmat emergency response / decontamination §
	Responder safety and health §
	Occupational health & safety

(Table adapted from Keim [17, 21, 33]. Entries marked as § are adapted from CDC, 2011 [101])
Source: Permission granted by Elsevier [19]

Resilience is the ability of a system exposed to hazards to resist, absorb, accommodate, and recover from the effects of a hazard in a timely and efficient manner. Examples of "resilience capacity" applied to disasters include economic, human, informational, and administrative resources for applying **absorptive**, **adaptive**, and **transformative capacities** used after the disaster occurs [34, 35]. This is comparable to **response capacity** for disasters that typically include operational and logistical resources such as facilities, personnel, equipment, supplies, transportation, and communications. Within this application, these capacities for resilience are resources for improving response and recovery. In this sense, resilience is simply a sub-component of capacity for response and recovery. And as such, it measures the rate at which the system exposed to hazards can resist, absorb, accommodate, and recover. Later in this book, we apply the concepts of capability and capacity for disaster planning and gap analysis in Chapter 9 (Capability-Based Planning), Chapter 16 (Planning Assumptions), and Chapter 19 (Gap Analysis).

4.4 Capability-Based Planning As Part of an Integrated Emergency Preparedness Program

As mentioned in Section 4.2, the ADEPT™ planning wheel represents a standardized approach for *planning* the disaster-related core capabilities that integrate with the US National Preparedness System (a standardized process for *accomplishing* disaster-related core capabilities). As such, the ADEPT™ planning wheel represents a standardized system for capability-based planning designed to inform modern preparedness systems (applied to any mission area).

Considering that the US National Preparedness System is simply a modified version of the Deming cycle for quality control, the ADEPT™ planning wheel can be used with any operation or system where the Deming cycle is applicable. Uses include most business operations, not merely emergency management.

4.5 Implementation of a Preparedness Plan

Activities included in the preparedness plan are then implemented. These activities may include many projects, programs, policies, and procedures for achieving or sustaining

Table 4.4. Elements of an emergency preparedness program

- risk assessment
- emergency planning
- training and education
- early warning systems
- specialized communication systems
- databases and information management systems
- inventory and resource management systems
- resource stocks
- emergency exercises
- population protection systems
- incident management systems

preparedness. Similar to the "eleven E's of emergency preparedness" in Table 3.1, Table 4.4 lists some of the most common functional elements of an emergency preparedness program [18].

4.6 Monitoring and Evaluation

Procedures are put in place to monitor and evaluate how an integrated preparedness program is implemented and what needs to be done to improve it. **Monitoring and evaluation** (M&E) are used to assess the performance of projects, programs, and actions set up by organizations. **Monitoring** is a continuous assessment based on the progress of ongoing activities. **Evaluation** is an examination concerning the relevance, quality, and impact of activities (usually performed at the end of an operational period). In other words, monitoring measures the inputs and outputs of activities, and evaluation measures objectives' outcomes. (See Chapter 22 for a detailed discussion of these procedures.)

Regardless of the subject, most programs are monitored using some form of **systems analysis**. Process analysis is the study of a process by mathematical means to define its goals and accomplish them most efficiently. As introduced in Chapter 3, program management applies processes and abilities to achieve long-term objectives, usually within mutually-agreed-upon resource parameters.

Like any program expected to produce an intended outcome, the quality of a preparedness program must also be managed to reduce uncertainty and improve its likelihood of success. Preparedness programs should be monitored regularly, with the preparedness plan itself serving as the standard. But of course, monitoring is not enough. This performance data is collected to define, measure, analyze, improve, and control for adverse variability among the preparedness program activities. The inputs (i.e., resources) and outputs (i.e., activities and deliverables) of the preparedness program are evaluated for critical indicators of performance, including timeliness, completeness, efficiency, and quality (e.g., stakeholder satisfaction). A preparedness program's outcomes are typically evaluated in terms of the effectiveness of meeting specific operational objectives or strategic goals.

In comparison to program monitoring, **evaluation** is an assessment concerning the relevance, effectiveness, and efficiency of specific objectives. Evaluation is used to measure short-, medium-, and long-term outcomes and guide future efforts.

4.7 Questions for Discussion

1. The terms "preparedness" and "planning" are sometimes mistakenly used interchangeably. Compare and contrast preparedness and planning in terms of strategy and tactics.
2. Describe the primary goal of plans written for each of the five mission areas (e.g., prevention, protection, mitigation, response, and recovery).

Questions for Discussion

Chapter

5 Eight Principles of Effective Planning

5.1 Learning Objectives

Upon completion of the chapter, the reader can:

1. Define the following terms and phrases:

    *   Activation
    *   Approach
    *   Assumption-based planning
    *   Black swans
    *   Community-based
    *   Delphi method
    *   Demobilization
    *   Efficacy
    *   End-user
    *   Facilitator
    *   Group facilitation
    *   Incident manager
    *   Job action sheets
    *   Measures of effectiveness
    *   Measures of efficiency
    *   Measures of success
    *   Memorandums of understanding
    *   Mutual aid agreements
    *   Partnership of equals
    *   Planning assumptions
    *   Points of contact
    *   Position
    *   Principles
    *   Satisfaction
    *   Social vulnerability index maps
    *   Townhall meeting
    *   Usability.

2. List eight principles of effective planning described by the mnemonic, "TARGET-UP:"

    *   Targeted to the need
    *   Accurately informed
    *   Realistic
    *   Goal-oriented

- Efficient
- Time-based
- Usable
- Position-centric.

3. Describe plan usability in terms of effectiveness, efficiency, satisfaction, and freedom from risk.

5.2 Principles for Effective Outcomes

Principles are treated as *fundamental truths* that are the foundation for a chain of reasoning. These principles are often applied as a general scientific theorem across a wide variety of fields and disciplines. **Approaches** are ways of applying these basic principles intended to improve the likelihood of success.

As illustrated in Table 1.1, **measures of effectiveness** describe the extent to which operations accomplish the intended outcomes. Thus, practical planning principles represent the foundation for accomplishing the intended outcomes of group deliberation and the written plan. Approaches for effective planning represent the methodology used for applying these principles.

The following are eight principles for effective planning, here represented by the mnemonic, "TARGET-UP.":

- Targeted to the need
- Accurately informed
- Realistic
- Goal-oriented
- Efficient
- Time-based
- Usable
- Position-centric.

5.3 Principle #1: Effective Plans Are Targeted to Meet the Need

The first principle for effective planning involves *targeting the plan to fit the need*. More information is necessary to target the plan for the appropriate end-user. First, "Is there a need for overarching strategy, or tactical detail, or an operational-level mix of the two?" Second, "Are the end-users comprised of leaders, or workers, or both?" And finally, "If this is an operational-level plan, then which emergency management mission area is involved (e.g., prevention, protection, mitigation, response, or recovery)?"

It is important to note that, in modern paradigms, we prepare for each of these disaster mission areas individually (compared to the old view of preparedness as a free-standing phase upon itself). Older models of preparedness also call for an "all-hazard" approach, preparing for all hazards – in all phases of the disaster cycle. These programs are prepared to respond to all hazards. But in the real world, most plans are (by necessity) more closely aligned with hazard likelihood and related justifications for public spending. For example, one may (reasonably) expect to find few mentions of snow removal in the "all-hazard" plans of tropical islands, and few plans for hurricane recovery in land-locked northern latitudes. When we unexpectedly discover such mentions, the logic of this approach comes into question.

> "All-hazard plans are so 'last year'"
> – Said Everyone

More recent preparedness approaches utilize risk assessments to guide interventions targeted to each specific mission area of the disaster cycle. For example, the prevention of flood-related mortality involves specific capabilities related to meteorological forecasting, land-use regulation, and floodplain management. On the contrary, the prevention of industrial chemical disasters involves entirely different capabilities like engineering controls, environmental monitoring, and hazard elimination/substitution. These both represent hazard-specific, not all-hazard approaches. During the response phase of the disaster cycle, preparedness activities should consider an all-hazard approach [18]. In emergency response, the uncertainty of hazard incidence and impact is overcome using a capability-based approach that facilitates an immediate and effective response, regardless of the causative hazard. We discuss this capability-based approach in more detail in Chapter 6, "The 02C3 Approach to Effective Planning."

5.4 Case Study: All-Hazard Planning in the South Pacific

In 2000, I was involved in assessing medical capabilities for Pacific island nations. This assessment included an inventory of healthcare resource capacity (e.g., facilities, equipment, supplies, and staffing) and an analysis of managerial and procedural capacity, as evidenced by the review of pertinent emergency operations plans.

On this occasion, Gary (a good friend and CDC senior public health advisor) and I had traveled to a remote tropical island located near the equator in the Pacific Ocean. We had spent the day touring the hospital, where we also obtained a copy of their newly-completed hospital disaster plan. After dinner, we had each retired to our respective hotel rooms and began our plan reviews. It all started seemingly normal. The title was ok. Also expectedly, the list of department heads and their signatures all graced the beginning of the hospital plan that characteristically started with general procedures and then, about ten pages later, began to explain hazard-specific actions.

And then I stopped reading. "What?" I laughed. I then grabbed up the plan and headed for the door. As I turned the corner, I could see Gary walking toward me outside in the hall. He was laughing too. We both read about the same speed because he had just read the same passage and was also coming to find me. On page twenty-five, there was a (rather nicely written) plan for snow removal at the hospital! A snow removal plan for a hospital that does not require indoor heating due to the year-round tropical climate. "Snow removal!" we both yelled nearly simultaneously in the hallway as we laughed.

"How did this happen?" you may ask. After reading further, we were able to discover that whoever had "written" the hospital plan must have grown tired of so much cutting and pasting and had failed to remove identifiers that named the hospital as one located along the Mississippi River in Minnesota! Later, the island hospital plan even included an annex related to a nuclear power plant (the closest nuclear facility to us was over 5,000 miles away).

While humorous, we can also appreciate the seriousness of a plan that is not targeted to meet the stakeholders' needs when it is most critically needed. There appear to be several factors that contributed to this result. The first is related to the number of resources that are commonly needed to develop an effective plan. It is not surprising that small, isolated, and under-funded hospitals would seek a shortcut. It is also not surprising that such a mistake was not identified early on during the planning process since the planning process itself should be targeted to the need. Here the perceived "need" was the need to be compliant with the hospital accreditation standards that require an emergency operations plan (without stipulations of quality or measures of its effectiveness). My friend and US Coast Guard colleague, Dr. Paul, later named this a "compliance plan" – when a plan is written primarily with the intent to comply with a requirement, rather than ensuring or improving safety. For this reason, the process of planning is paramount to successful execution. In effect, the planning is more important than the plan.

> "The process of planning is more important than the written document that results"
>
> – Erik Auf der Heide

The process of iterative stakeholder negotiations regarding commitments for cooperation is crucial for developing a **common operating picture**. A common operating picture facilitates collaborative planning and combined execution and assists all stakeholders in achieving **situational awareness**.

In this sense, the plan is like a contract, and the stakeholders are the negotiators. With each iteration, stakeholders hear their partners' intended actions and commitments and then react to align their activities to meet the common operational objectives. The planning process itself is thus the first step of quality control before subsequent plan communication and dissemination.

> "Everyone has a plan, until they get punched in the face"
>
> – Mike Tyson

5.5 Principle #2: Effective Plans Are Accurately Informed

The second principle for effective planning is that the process must be accurately informed. Planning must be based upon valid assumptions regarding disaster risk, including probabilistic estimations of hazards, exposure, impact, and capabilities. Unfortunately, the availability of such "hard data" is relatively limited for non-material assets, such as the public health and safety of a population.

RAND defines **planning assumptions** are "an assertion about some characteristic of the future that underlies the current operations or plans of an organization" [36, p. 5]. Unforeseen surprises (i.e., **black swans**) can often be traced to the failure of an assumption that the organization's leadership did not anticipate or had "forgotten" it was making. To quote former US Secretary of Defense Donald Rumsfeld during his explanation of risk analysis,

... there are "known knowns"; there are things we know we know. We also know there are "known unknowns"; that is to say, we know there are some things we do not know. But there are also "unknown unknowns" – the ones we don't know we don't know. And if one looks throughout the history of our country and other free countries, it is the latter category that tends to be the difficult one. [37]

> "We don't always know what we don't know"
> – Donald Rumsfeld

Figure 17.2 further details how a hazard-impact matrix fails to take into consideration these so-called unknown unknowns (i.e., "black swans"). These events represent previously unrecognized hazards and threats – in other words, hazards with an incidence erroneously estimated as "no probability" (either by commission or omission) and are therefore not included in the hazard-impact matrix.

Assumption-based planning is a tool for identifying as many assumptions underlying an organization's plans as possible and bringing those assumptions explicitly into the planning process. Explicit assumptions are clear, precise, and specific. They characteristically lack ambiguity. Implicit assumptions are not stated and may go undetected. If implicit assumptions are wrong, this can prevent successful outcomes. Assumption-based planning typically identifies these assumptions and then determines and tests their criticality in the plan [38].

Beyond the complications associated with assumptions that must be made in the face of uncertainty, there are also severe challenges in obtaining historical evidence to base decision-making. "The fundamental difficulty in disaster risk assessment is determining the frequency of hazard occurrence since historical information is not available on all kinds of past incidents" [39]. Furthermore, "evaluating the severity of the consequences (impact) is also often quite difficult for immaterial assets." Thus, "best-educated opinions and available statistics are the primary sources of information" [39]. Nevertheless, qualitative or semi-quantitative risk assessment can produce such information so that the primary risks are easy to understand and that the risk management decisions may be prioritized.

The most relevant information sources and techniques should be used when collecting information that informs disaster planning. Sources of information may include the following [1, 40]:

- Applicable authorities and statutes.
- Pre-existing disaster plans.
- Risk assessments, including intentional threats and unintentional hazards.
- Planning guidance that is pertinent to the jurisdiction, hazard, and disaster phase.
- After action reports of performance during prior simulations and real events.
- Hazard and **social vulnerability index maps** for the geographical location or jurisdiction.
- **Points of contact** and contact information for stakeholder organizations.
- **Mutual aid agreements** and **memorandums of understanding**.
- Reports of pertinent practice and relevant experience.
- Relevant published literature.
- The results of public or private consultations (e.g., **townhall meetings**, contracts).

5.6 Principle #3: Effective Plans Are Realistic

Plans must adhere to a third principle, realism. My good friend and CDC colleague, Erik Auf der Heide, has pointed out that planning assumptions must also be based upon "valid assumptions about human behavior" [14, p. 35]. We must plan according to how people *will* behave, not how people *should* behave. Our plans must offer realistic solutions based upon actual capabilities, not planned, or predicted, or hoped-for capabilities of the future. When we write a plan today, it should be based upon today's capability – as though we would have to implement the plan *immediately*. The ends and means must be realistic and achievable according to current capabilities (not a future target). Otherwise, there is a risk of implementing a plan that is not entirely correct – when effectiveness is thwarted by yet-unrealized accomplishments (and therefore, false assumptions of capability). Plan deliberation can proceed to surprisingly advanced levels before some groups can identify that particular objectives or activities may be unrealistic to consider in the plan.

For example, during one hospital disaster planning session in 2002, I witnessed plan stakeholders identify chemical decontamination of patients as a core capability of the hospital. (It was included in a related grant ☺.) Once identified as a capability, the stakeholders worked together to identify a series of related strategic and operational objectives accomplished by detailed activities. They performed all of this planning before concluding that the capability did not exist because they could not identify any staff member appropriately trained to perform the task. Was this time wasted? I do not believe that it was. Here is my reasoning. The group collectively identified a gap in their capability in advance (when it is much easier to rectify through mutual aid agreements or external humanitarian assistance) than ad hoc decisions made during the event.

Realistic objectives are considered one of the five "SMART" elements of effective objectives [41]. (Objective-based planning is discussed in greater detail in Chapter 8.) Realistic plans state what results can realistically be achieved, given available resources. Realism is also an essential requirement when managers seek to monitor, evaluate, and control subsequent operations according to the measures of success stated in the plan. It may be tempting for stakeholders to write a plan where capabilities or capacity are overstated in a well-intended attempt at "encouragement" or "optimism." In these cases, planners may feel compelled to state unrealistic outcomes with the consideration that accomplishing a significant portion of a lofty goal may be preferable to accomplishing all of a less ambitious one. The opposite is true. Specific and measurably realistic goals provide incident managers with a widely-agreed-upon scale to monitor and evaluate emergency operations progress. These goals should represent the stakeholders' realistic expectations that are to be imparted to the incident manager. Plans must describe what we *will* do, not what we *could* or *should* do.

5.7 Principle #4: Effective Plans Are Goal-Oriented

The fourth principle for effective planning is goal orientation. The plan format should be a statement of broad goals that are accomplished through corresponding actions. This format is intended to contrast with other plan formats that may involve a chronological (time-based) listing of expected actions without outcome or intent statements.

Goals are used to direct actions because while the actions required to accomplish a task may change over time or location, the goal is a much more stable representation of the plan's intended capability. Goals allow for a range of activity options to be considered and implemented with a synergistic effect. Goals also form the coordinating connection between strategy and operations. Goals also help to prevent "mission creep" – superfluous activities that expand the workload but not operational effectiveness in terms of outcome.

Goal-oriented planning is fundamentally objective-based. As introduced in Chapter 1, Drucker's model for management by objectives is based upon this same principle of goal setting as a means for quality control [42]. Management by objectives is a system for comparing actual performance with expected (or planned) performance. Goal-oriented planning describes measures of success – the intended state of being when the outcome is achieved. Goals and objectives are, therefore, always a description of a successful outcome. Whenever I facilitate planning sessions, I encourage stakeholders to (silently) preface their statements of strategic goals or operational objectives with the phrase, "We know we're successful when . . ." followed by a statement of the goal. For example, "We know we are successful when . . .," "All nurses have adequate access to US Occupational Safety and Health Administration (OSHA)-approved personal protective equipment (PPE)." The resultant objective is specific and measurable.

5.8 Principle #5: Effective Plans Are Efficient

The fifth principle of effective planning is efficiency. Planning is a labor-intensive under-taking. It requires the participation and coordination of multiple organizations across different jurisdictions. More extensive organizational or **community-based** planning sessions routinely involve 30–50 stakeholder participants. The importance of efficiency is magnified when considering the opportunity cost associated with one hour of disaster planning as a plenary.

Each hour spent together planning as a group utilizes thirty-to-fifty personnel hours that could be otherwise allocated to preparedness. Thus, one day spent planning could potentially waste 240–400 personnel hours. It is also frustrating for stakeholders to partici-pate in planning sessions that are not operated efficiently. **Group facilitation** is a helpful technique for moderating group discussions and decision-making during planning. Adequate preparation and promptness are critical characteristics for stakeholder participa-tion. Insufficient or overly aggressive moderation and facilitation can also hamper effi-ciency. Language and cultural barriers may also contribute to a less efficient planning process. Finally, to be a fair broker of the public trust, community-based planning must also encourage professional partners' collaboration while remaining committed to a **part-nership of equals** that also serve public partners and produce valuable outcomes for the entire community [43, 44]. "Official" organizations should be encouraged to maximize the efficiency of planning by listening and learning about the role of non-traditional partners (as compared to time spent describing agency-specific procedures or the familiar refrain of "This is the way that we've always done it").

5.9 Principle #6: Effective Plans Are Time-Based

The sixth principle for effective planning is that objectives are time-based, meaning an exact deadline or expected timeframe for completion. In the absence of time duration estimates, it is impossible to predict plan efficiency and resource allocation (e.g., personnel, funding, materials). Without measures of time duration, estimations of capacity rates also become less relevant for ensuring adequate capability.

However, it should also be noted that, in most cases, it is quite tricky to predict the exact chronological or sequential order that many plan activities will be implemented according to any given scenario. For this reason, time-based planning seeks to measure the time duration needed to accomplish an objective (or each of its associated activities). It does not specify the exact timing for the initiation of each time-based intervention. Multiple, cross-cutting activities typically begin and end simultaneously with **activation** and **demobilization** of the incident response.

5.10 Principle #7: Effective Plans Are Usable

Any intervention (including planning) is influenced by the effectiveness, efficiency, degree of satisfaction, and "freedom from risk" perceived among participants [45, 46]. To be usable, the planning process must not only be effective and efficient, but the community must also perceive them to have a value that outweighs potential social, economic, environmental, or health risks.

And while effectiveness research is commonplace in other public health areas, there have been very few studies of intervention effectiveness related to disasters. Despite the repeated urging of public health leadership, disaster epidemiology remains chiefly concerned with etiological rather than evaluative hypotheses [47, 48].

Efficacy is a measure of an intervention's performance under controlled circumstances (compared to effectiveness, which is a measure of performance under "real-world" conditions) [49].

Measures of effectiveness relate to the quality of outcomes. In comparison, **measures of efficiency** are related to the quality of performance (usually as a rate). Effectiveness describes the degree to which objectives are achieved. In simplest terms, it involves "doing the right things." In comparison, efficiency describes a level of performance that uses the least number of resources (e.g., time, people, money) to achieve these objectives. It involves "doing things right." For planning to be successful, it must be both effective and efficient. Such operations provide a baseline for the scalable development of policies and procedures that create short-, medium-, and long-term impact.

Besides effectiveness and efficiency, an intervention's usability is also influenced by the degree of satisfaction and freedom from risk perceived among participants. The most usable interventions engender a high degree of community satisfaction with the *process* (e.g., consensus-based decision-making) and the *content* (e.g., evacuation or shelter-in-place). **Satisfaction** is a customer-focused measure of quality. In simple terms, it involves "ensuring value" for the project participant. Participant value is a function of the relative risk of participation (i.e., economic, social, environmental, and health) compared to the benefit of participation [23].

Thus, the usability of an intervention depends on perceived freedom from risk on behalf of the participants [45]. While the risk of participating in planning workshops may appear negligibly related to economic, health, or environmental threats, some participants (especially those in positions of authority or responsibility) may perceive a significant social risk related to their attendance and engagement in planning workshops (especially for events of high public interest). Social risks include the potential to give the appearance that one (or one's agency) is: (1) poorly informed; (2) poorly suited to perform a task for which one is responsible; (3) overly cooperative with a rival group; or (4) unwilling to commit responsibility for activities identified in the plan. The most usable planning processes take into consideration economic, social, environmental, and health risks that may influence the full range of public and private community members [27].

5.11 Principle #8: Effective Plans Are Position-centric

The eighth principle for effective plans is based upon the need for instructions targeted to the appropriate **position** of the **end-user**. The end-users of strategic plans typically differ from those of operational and tactical plans. The role of organizational leadership (chief executives, public information officers, and incident managers) typically involves implementing strategic goals. Whereas the role of organizational workers (e.g., line managers, operations staff, subject matter experts, support staff) typically involves implementing plan operations and the more detailed tactical activities of the plan.

As I often state, while facilitating such planning sessions, "Plans are best written by those people that actually 'do' the job." Plans must also be accurately informed so that decision-making is based upon the best evidence (not merely the most prevalent opinion in the room). Thus, like the **Delphi method**, also used for **group-based decision-making**, the accuracy of group-based planning depends on the subject matter expertise (e.g., knowledge, skills, abilities, and experience) of the participants. Like the Delphi method, in group planning, it is essential to take measures that prevent some participants' authority, personality, or reputation from dominating others in the process. In planning, the quality of this process is controlled through close facilitation by a moderator. A facilitator's use helps to encourage the free expression of opinions, open critique, and admission of errors when revising earlier judgments.

The sources of subject matter expertise related to strategic planning often differ from that needed for detailed operational planning. In some cases, both strategic and tactical thinkers are needed. However, in many cases, plans written with the appropriate level of operational and strategic levels of detail are best written by workers and managers (rather than chief officers and executives). During planning sessions, organizations may be tempted to send representatives to the plan-writing process that does not have a comprehensive perspective of the organization's operations. Typically, these are junior staff assigned to "represent" the agency in multi-sectoral/multi-organizational planning (because they are more easily "spared" from routine business functions). This approach results in the least senior staff writing a plan that speaks for the entire organization in a time of high risk and uncertainty.

Conversely, plans written by those that are too senior tend to lack the tactical level of detail necessary to accomplish effective operations. It is necessary to have a mix of leadership and staff involved in the planning process. It is also necessary to target plan outputs (e.g., activities and responsibilities) to the appropriate audience level. Leaders tend to focus on their objectives. Workers tend to focus on activities. The **incident manager** controls worker activities in support of leadership objectives according to **measures of success** (e.g., effectiveness and efficiency). Therefore, both the planning process and the plan must be targeted to address the end-users' strategic and operational needs.

Finally, it is a simple but not infrequent mistake to write plans based upon the individual people (compared to the professional position) that perform the activity. Most would agree that a clear statement of responsibility is critical to effective emergency operations. And yet, on close examination, surprisingly few plans assign direct responsibility to specific tasks. In many cases, this is either implied, assigned only at the organizational level, or not addressed. In some cases, the plans may assign the responsibility to a specific person named in the plan. This practice is considered unacceptable because that person may or may not be currently employed, scheduled, and available during the full extent of all emergency operations. Therefore, considerations should be given for staffing coverage based upon the capability and capacity described in the operations plan. Staffing is usually accomplished by developing a daily incident action plan that allocates resources for each task. The incident action plan then includes staffing arrangements that are based upon job or position requirements. These requirements are most often detailed in the form of tactical-level **job action sheets** or employee **position descriptions** in the case of full-time emergency responders.

5.12 Questions for Discussion

1. Compare efficiency and effectiveness as measures of process and outcome.
2. Discuss the importance of having the "right person" involved in planning.
3. Describe the characteristics of a plan targeted to meet the informational needs of leaders, as compared to workers.
4. Describe the characteristics of a plan targeted to meet the informational needs of disaster victims, as compared to workers.

Chapter

The O2C3 Approach to Effective Planning

6.1 Learning Objectives

Upon completion of the chapter, the reader can:

1. Define the following terms and phrases:
   - Compliance
   - Consensus
   - Key performance indicator (KPI)
   - Knowledge skills and abilities (KSA)
   - O2C3 planning
   - Standard model
   - Standard of practice.

2. Describe the five approaches included in O2C3 planning:
   - Operational level
   - Objective-based
   - Capability-based
   - Consensus-based
   - Compliance with strategy.

6.2 Five Approaches to Effective Planning

The "**O2C3**" **planning** combines five approaches for effective planning (e.g., operational-level, objective-based, capability-based, consensus-based, and compliant with population norms and regulations) [13, 21, 25, 28, 33, 50, 51]. This book describes the O2C3 model as a single paradigm for unifying modern planning and coordination theories.

6.3 Operational Approach to Planning

As introduced in Chapter 1, operational planning is a subset of strategic planning [1]. Operational plans describe short-term ways of achieving operational objectives and explain how (or what portion of) a strategic plan is placed into operation during a given period. Operational plans describe the tactical details (i.e., the "who, what, and where" that will be accomplished) and link these tactics to strategy (i.e., the "why" that describes a goal or outcome).

As discussed in Chapter 1, Fayol described operations as a group of processes implemented by an organization according to a strategy [2]. Management of emergency operations includes designing and maintaining an incident command system in which individuals are working together in groups to accomplish emergency objectives. Simply stated, emergency management is a system used to accomplish the emergency goals of a population. Emergency managers are responsible for the development, maintenance, and improvement of this system.

Thus, operational planning is one of the five critical functions of emergency managers (e.g., *planning*, organizing, staffing, leading, and controlling) [1]. Emergency managers use operational plans to establish a previously agreed-upon **standard model** against which future operations may be compared. According to measurable indicators of performance and outcome, emergency managers use operational plans to benchmark key accomplishments. Operational plans must, therefore, be oriented toward measurable performance and outcomes. They must clearly describe the intended state of accomplishment and the measures for its success. In simple terms, operational plans describe the "ends" (i.e., strategy) and then detail the "means" (i.e., operations and tactics) for reaching them.

6.4 Objective-Based Approach to Planning

An objective (i.e., goal) is the object of an effort. It is the aim or desired result of work activity. Objectives describe a projected situation – a desired endpoint in some sort of assumed development [28]. As such, objective-based planning is based on goal setting and outcomes. Objectives describe the parameters of a successful outcome that are specific, measurable, attainable, realistic, and time-based [41]. These criteria help identify and describe **key performance indicators** (e.g., **knowledge, skills, and abilities, KSAs**) that reflect the successful accomplishment of these objectives given the current resource constraints (e.g., capability and capacity).

Goal setting promotes long-term vision and short-term motivation. It focuses on the acquisition of knowledge and helps to organize resources. Knowing what one wants to achieve then makes it obvious what to focus on and improve. Objectives ensure that participants have a clear awareness of what they must do to achieve (or help achieve) an outcome.

> "What gets measured, gets managed"
> – Peter Drucker

If our objectives are clear, we are not sidetracked by ad hoc, non-essential suggestions during plan-writing – this clarity in goal-setting results in efficient planning with less variability (i.e., less uncertainty). If our objectives are clear, we are not sidetracked during emergency response when unforeseen "black swan" events may preclude one course of action while sparing other alternative activities that may also accomplish the same outcome – this clarity of intent results in effective planning with less variability (i.e., less uncertainty).

> "The best laid plans of mice and men often go awry"
> – Robert Burns

6.5 Capability-Based Approach to Planning

Unfortunately, objective-based planning is too often based upon minimal assumptions. No matter how a project is planned, misfortunes may still occur. Thus, when used alone, the objective-based approach may imply a false degree of certainty regarding the disaster hazard or threat that is not attainable.

In addition to limiting the range of solutions, objective-based planning often generates a list without establishing priorities [52]. It is therefore necessary to include a planning approach that addresses this degree of uncertainty regarding our ability to predict disaster risk. Capability-based planning allows for more flexible emergency operations plans (EOPs) to be developed that address a myriad of unpredictable contingencies.

A capability is defined as the "ability to achieve a desired operational effect under specified standards and conditions through combinations of means and ways to perform a set of activities" [53]. Capabilities are inventoried based upon the activities required. Once the required capability inventory is defined, the most cost-effective and efficient options to satisfy the requirements are sought [54, 55]. Capability-based planning involves "Planning under uncertainty to provide capabilities suitable for a wide range of modern-day challenges and circumstances while working within an economic framework that necessitates choice" [55, p. xi].

Capability-based planning focuses on goals and outcomes and encourages innovative approaches and processes. Capabilities also provide the common framework used for relating and comparing disparate elements of an incident command system.

6.6 Consensus-Based Approach to Planning

Consensus-based decision-making is a group decision-making process that seeks the agreement of most participants and resolves or mitigates the objections of the minority to achieve the most agreeable decision. **Consensus** is defined in terms of a general agreement and the process of getting to such an agreement [13]. Consensus-based decision-making is thus concerned primarily with that process.

Consensus aims to be inclusive, participatory, cooperative, and egalitarian [28]. Consensus-based decision-making seeks agreement and resolves or mitigates the minority's objections to achieve the most agreeable decision. Consensus-based decision-making serves to incorporate community socio-economic and cultural input in all aspects of the process, encouraging stakeholdership and commitment. The process results in equitable partnerships that require the sharing of power, resources, attribution, results, and knowledge, as well as a mutual appreciation of each partner's knowledge and skills.

Consensus-based planning allows the various stakeholders to negotiate this new and less familiar paradigm for social and professional interaction before the disaster response. The written plan is only one outcome of the planning process. Consensus-based planning itself provides a significant opportunity to build partnerships and encourage stakeholdership. The planning process is also a way for stakeholders to learn the plan and to share in decision-making. The plan should be viewed as a contract that documents the negotiation among all stakeholders.

6.7 Compliance-Based Approach to Planning

Effective plans are also compliant with international, national, regional, and local strategies. Compliant plans conform to a rule, such as a specification, policy, standard, or law. All plans must comply with existing laws and all pertinent policies, procedures, guidelines, and recommendations related to the action.

Compliance recognizes the legal mandate, responsibility, and constraints of the organization and its correlating role with other organizations and other incident command systems. Compliant plans also conform to a standardized organizational structure that is reproducible and recognizable across sectors.

In addition to community added socio-economic and cultural input added through consensus-based planning, external legal and regulatory inputs are also integrated into the plan.

Finally, plans must be compliant with local cultural norms. Particular attention should be paid to local variations in these social and cultural norms so that the plans reflect the individuals' real intent or organizations that they are intended to serve.

Plan for consequences, not merely compliance

6.8 Questions for Discussion

1. Describe how objectives help to lessen the variability associated with operations.
2. Describe how consensus helps to lessen the variability associated with compliance.
3. Give one example of the following situations:
   a. A stakeholder has adequate resources (i.e., capacity) to complete an objective, but still cannot do so.
   b. A stakeholder has adequate knowledge and skills to complete an activity, but still cannot do so.
4. Describe potential (social, economic, political, environmental, and health) "risks" that may be associated with a stakeholder's participation in community-based planning.

Operational Planning

7.1 Learning Objectives

Upon completion of the chapter, the reader can:

1. Define the following terms and phrases:
   - Anecdotal
   - Decision tree
   - Empirical
   - Evidence-based decision-making
   - Modeling
   - Operations research
   - Probabilistic analysis
   - Process control
   - Quantitative analysis
   - Simulation
   - Task analysis.

7.2 Operations Management

Operations management is the business practice of creating the highest possible efficiency level. Operations are designed to convert materials and labor into goods and services as efficiently as possible to maximize an organization's profit (or public impact). In this book, operations management includes designing and controlling the production of services related to emergencies (i.e., emergency management), specifically related to health.

> "Planning means both to assess the future and make provision for it"
>
> – Henri Fayol

7.3 Operations As a System

As introduced in Chapter 1, systems are groups of processes that transform inputs (i.e., resources) into outputs and outcomes (i.e., objectives). As also discussed in Chapter 1, operations consist of a group of processes (i.e., groups of activities) implemented according to a particular objective strategy. Figure 7.1 depicts how processes are a means to coordinate

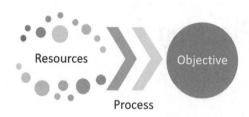

Figure 7.1 Operations as a system with three components: resources, processes, and objectives

inputs (e.g., personnel, equipment, time, funding) that accomplish the intended outcome (e.g., shelter, nutrition, hydration, and health). The figure also represents the function of operations as a system of inputs, outputs, and outcomes.

During emergencies, most incident command systems characteristically include six major functional areas: command, operations, planning, logistics, intelligence/investigations, and finance/administration [56]. As a primary function of incident management, emergency operations represent a set of processes (i.e., activities), implemented according to a plan (i.e., strategy), that use inputs (i.e., resources) to create outputs (i.e., activities) that accomplish safe and healthy outcomes (i.e., goals or objectives). The emergency manager's role is to utilize an incident command system (ICS) to plan, organize, staff, lead, and control that group of processes that comprise emergency operations to accomplish the objectives of the emergency operations plan (EOP), while using the least number of resources.

EOPs describe the real business – the "raison d'être" of the incident command system. They are not intended to be administrative, intelligence-related, or logistic plans that describe the activities' support. They are also not a prevention, protection, and mitigation plan intended to be completed *before* the hazard threatens or occurs. EOPs describe and assign detailed operational activities that accomplish the primary objective of protecting lives, health, and property once the hazard is *imminent* or *after* it has already occurred.

Like objective-based planning, operational plans also enforce a certain degree of accountability and responsibility for these actions' successful performance. The development, maintenance, and improvement of operational plans establish a process for plan stakeholders to justify actions or decisions. It is often no coincidence that many bad managers (and bad employees) tend to shy away from plans and planning. Operational-level plans add a layer of detail that requires accountability from management and workers (and from government and the community!)

Operational level detail also allows for quality improvement regarding **process control** and cost accounting for individual activities, operational objectives, or strategic goals. Process inputs and outputs may be monitored and evaluated for efficiency, according to the plan activities. According to the plan objectives, indicators of short-, medium-, and long-term process outcomes may also be evaluated for effectiveness.

7.4 Operations Research

When considered a system, emergency operations (like all business operations) may then be evaluated using the scientific method, the basis for modern research. **Operations research** is the "application of scientific methods to the study of alternatives in a problem situation, with a view of obtaining a quantitative basis for arriving at the best solution" [1]. The emphasis is on the use of quantitative data, goals, and determination of the best course of action for achieving those goals. Operations research has six key characteristics as follows [1]: (1) it is based upon representative models; (2) it is based upon measurable goals; (3) it incorporates controllable variables; (4) it represents the process in mathematical terms; (5) it quantifies the variables as much as possible; and (6) it supplements unavailable data with mathematical and statistical devices as the probability of a given situation. These characteristics allow for the **probabilistic analysis** of algorithms for various courses of action that lend themselves to **decision trees**. A decision tree is a tree-like model of decisions and possible consequences, including chance event outcomes, resource costs, and utility. Decision trees are commonly used in operational research. This research includes decision analysis to help identify a strategy most likely to reach a goal.

There has been a chronic and long-standing paucity of operations research related to disasters, primarily related to health. In the US, nationally led calls for enabling rapid and sustainable operations research applied to public health have yet to gain fiscal attention [47, 48].

Operations research requires the level of operational detail necessary to evaluate the effectiveness and efficiency of process control methods used for individual activities, operational objectives, or strategic goals. For example, it is possible to monitor and evaluate operations' progress when the plan itself is based upon a detailed description of operations (e.g., inputs, outputs, and outcomes).

EOPs may also be monitored and evaluated according to measures of quality that involve these same inputs, outputs, and outcomes (i.e., resources, activities, and objectives). Individual tactics may be monitored and evaluated according to process indicators (e.g., time, materials, and human resources). According to the plan strategy, indicators of short-, medium-, and long-term outcomes may also be evaluated for effectiveness.

The operational level of detail in an EOP allows for **quantitative analysis** that further informs future decision-making. **Probabilistic analysis** is also used to refine EOPs by analyzing operational details (e.g., modeling, simulation, and activities during real events). Most emergency operations evaluations use **anecdotal**, as opposed to **practical** information derived by the scientific method. These empirical results of operations research are used to inform **evidence-based decision-making** during emergency operations.

7.5 Questions for Discussion

1. Describe the role of operational plans for ensuring the accountability of leadership.
2. Give an example of the inputs, outputs, and outcomes for making breakfast.
3. Compare quantitative analysis to qualitative analysis and give one example of each.

Objective-Based Planning

8.1 Learning Objectives

Upon completion of the chapter, the reader can:

1. Define the following terms and phrases:
   - Accountability
   - Channels of communication
   - Negotiation
   - Uncertainty.
2. List the four key benefits of objective-based planning.
3. Describe how objective-based planning improves accountability.
4. Describe how objective-based planning establishes channels of communication.
5. Describe how objective-based planning promotes plan negotiation.
6. List the five significant steps of management by objectives.
7. List Doran's SMART objectives.
8. Categorize the following statements as describing either an objective or an activity:
   - Serve the dinner.
   - The dinner is served.

8.2 Four Critical Benefits of Objective-Based Planning

There are four key benefits to objective-based planning: (1) reducing uncertainty; (2) improving accountability; (3) establishing channels of communication among stakeholders; and (4) promoting negotiation of the plan.

8.2.1 Objectives Reduce Uncertainty

Objective-based planning offers a means for reducing the **uncertainty** inherent in emergency operations. Plans describe purposeful actions intended to occur in the future [57]. As such, plans offer a course of action that is considered likely, but not sure to occur. The accomplishment of these actions is intended to result in a specific outcome. Variances in these actions' performance expectedly result in a lower degree of certainty, reproducibility, and transferability of the intended outcomes. Management is a tool used to improve the certainty that a given process produces the intended outcome (i.e., effectiveness) within the constraints of available resources (i.e., efficiency).

One of the defining elements of objective-based planning is the starting point of the timeline. Objective-based planning begins with a future goal and works backward to the present. Planners align future goals with a specific time of achievement. In comparison, issues-based planning (commonly used by the lay public) starts from the present and works toward the future. Issue-based plans are often used to organize short-term actions where certainty regarding outcomes (effectiveness) is less critical than certainty regarding process performance (i.e., efficiency) or constraints placed upon resources.

Swann has proposed that "Objective-based planning is the only rational approach to planning. An alternative is a laissez-faire approach that inevitably ends in chaos" [52, p. 38]. It has also been this author's experience in facilitating several hundred planning sessions worldwide that issue-based planning is an inefficient process for collaborative planning. While they usually tend to start well, the process becomes much more complicated when divergent opinions occur, and actions begin to cross-relate.

> A response (or exercise) without a plan is like a play without a script.

Issue-based planning fails to recognize that goals are also a tangible product of personal values. The individual's attitude, beliefs, and cultural background inform their goals. And while a group of individuals may begin at the same time working toward the future on the same issue, the outcome can become highly variable without some metric for completion. The mental construct of what that future outcome may look like is influenced by the attitude, beliefs, and cultural backgrounds of multiple individuals. The more complex the plan becomes (as it adds more stages and more individual perspectives), the higher the risk of uncertainty regarding plan outcome. I like to compare planning to the script of the play. You may be able to perform satisfactorily one night without a script. But repeatability is nearly impossible, and the audience experience is likely to vary each night remarkably. (Watch out for the thrown cabbage!)

8.2.2 Objectives Improve Accountability

With an established metric for success (e.g., objective), we may quantify progress and adjust the process to produce the desired outcome. Without clear objectives, monitoring and evaluation become anecdotal, focusing on short-term measures of the process (e.g., number of patients treated) compared to longer-term measures of outcome (e.g., change in case fatality rate).

Clearly stated objectives also assign responsibility for accomplishment. This responsibility is discussed, negotiated, and committed to during the planning process and then activated, monitored, and evaluated during plan execution. The **accountability** of plan stakeholders is a critical planning assumption that must be continuously monitored and evaluated. The collective effort's success depends on the ability of the individual stakeholders to accomplish their respective tasks. Objectives allow for the development of clearly stated roles and responsibilities. Objective-based plans provide incident managers with a pre-negotiated commitment of responsibilities that may then be used to guide accountability among the various plan stakeholders.

> "You can't manage what you can't measure"
> – Peter Drucker

8.2.3 Objectives Establish Channels of Communication

Objective-based planning brings together stakeholders for detailed discussions regarding collective efforts. Key issues are identified and then discussed with appropriate counterparts from other groups. Autocrats discuss strategy while their subordinates, the technocrats, discuss operations and tactics. Points of contact are identified, and relationships are developed.

As the emergency preparedness saying goes, "Better now than at 2 am when it's raining." In other words, it is better to talk now than during the emergency – which always seems to occur at the most inopportune time. And while that is easy to say, it is surprising how often that little attention is paid to establishing relationships that extend outside of the emergency operation itself. Most emergency managers recognize the value of knowing the person on the other end of the phone and their mindset before an emergency. And yet, I have attended numerous disasters where the points of contact and **communication channels** were not established in advance (particularly in the private health sector). I recall during one particular flood disaster response that I was involved in when the staff member of a federal disaster medical assistance team had the unenviable job of pulling together a telephone contact list of local healthcare providers during the disaster when most facilities were closed (before the Internet and cell phones were available). It was nearly midnight as they looked up from their hard copy spreadsheet and, for what seemed the tenth time, pondered aloud, "Why didn't we do this before?" Then, with a shrug of the shoulders, (a nurse from Arkansas) went back to establishing communication channels (in the middle of the night) where they did not previously exist (in North Dakota).

8.2.4 Objectives Facilitate Negotiation of the Plan

Negotiation of a plan is like the negotiation of a contract. Assumptions are stated upfront regarding the need. Plan stakeholders then identify goals and discuss potential courses of action to address this need by performing work. Finally, stakeholders negotiate and agree upon a mutually beneficial course of action that addresses the need. This process of negotiation often requires iteration. The steps of negotiation typically include the following five steps:

1. identification of needs,
2. brainstorming discussion of potential courses of action,
3. proposal of activities by responsible parties,
4. iterative discussion, followed by
5. self-commitment to perform the activity.

The resultant plan is, in effect, the contract that documents this mutual agreement among all stakeholders.

Dillard's "goals, plans, action" theory of interpersonal communication makes the following assumptions: individuals are predictable; goals are based on deeper values; and their behavior is intentional [57]. The theory posits a limited number of primary goals that drive all human plans and ultimately lead to action. With each of the goals, the individual intends to provide or obtain something to further their relationship with others. Goals thus represent a larger construct of social interaction that drives human behavior to collaborate. In essence, planning represents an alignment of these individual goals to comprise the collective mutually beneficial goals. Objective-based planning begins with a statement of the common goal. The attainment of this common goal implies the successful communication and negotiation of individual goals. For this reason, an objective-based approach to planning is preferable to an issue-based approach that does not inform the planning process regarding stakeholder attitude, beliefs, and values.

8.3 Management by Objectives

Management by objectives (MBO) is a strategic management model applied in business and emergency management. For business, MBO represents a standardized system used for both planning as well as performance management. At the time, Drucker's original model was considered innovative in that it was the first to include employee input into goal setting, measurement, and performance evaluation. There are five steps in MBO as follows: (1) review organizational goal; (2) set worker objective; (3) monitor progress; (4) evaluation; and (5) give a reward. Central to the concept of MBO is the alignment of organizational goals with worker objectives [42]. This collaborative approach to the managerial functions of planning and controlling the system allows for a more accurate alignment of individual goals with mutually beneficial goals of the collaborative. For this reason, MBO and its related versions represent the mainstay of most public and private systems used for strategic management.

8.4 Case Study: MBO As a Fundamental Principle of US Incident Command Systems

Management by objectives is one of the fourteen fundamental principles underpinning the US National Incident Management System (NIMS) (as the standardized incident command system) used in the United States. When applied to emergency operations, MBO involves the following activities [1]:

- establishing overarching incident objectives,
- developing strategies based on incident objectives,
- developing and issuing assignments, plans, procedures, and protocols,
- establishing specific, measurable objectives for target capabilities,
- directing efforts to attain capabilities in support of defined strategies, and
- documenting results to measure performance and facilitate corrective action.

In this model, emergency management convenes other stakeholders in advance of the disaster to perform planning functions for subsequent incidents. Once the disaster occurs, emergency management then reconvenes the stakeholders' system to collaborate in controlling (e.g., measuring and correcting) the process. Thus, MBO allows for the alignment of individual or agency goals with the collective's mutually beneficial goals through the emergency operations plan. Emergency managers use MBO to monitor and evaluate ongoing emergency operations to ensure the intended outcome as detailed in the emergency operations plan – a pre-negotiated commitment of responsibilities and resources among the various plan stakeholders.

8.5 SMART Objectives

Objectives require quantitative analysis. Reliable systems are needed to establish relevant objectives and monitor their degree of accomplishment in an objective way.

S-M-A-R-T is a mnemonic used in objective-based planning. It is a way of evaluating if the objectives that are being set are appropriate for the individual project. SMART criteria help us to write objectives according to quantifiable and reproducible terms. According to Drucker, a SMART objective is specific, measurable, *achievable*, *relevant*, and time-bound [42]. Doran further characterized "SMART" objectives as follows:

- Specific – Target a specific area for improvement.
- Measurable – Quantify an indicator of progress.
- *Assignable* – Specify who does it.
- *Realistic* – State what results can realistically be achieved, given the available resources.
- Time-bound – Specify when the result(s) can be achieved [41].

> "What gets measured, gets managed"
>
> – Peter Drucker

8.6 Writing SMART Objectives

For planning purposes, objectives describe the intended outcome using the *passive present tense* – to describe how the objective has been accomplished (e.g., "All assessments are completed," "100 shelters are available," "Information is provided," "Tarps are delivered").

One easy method for writing plan objectives in the proper tense is to preface the intended objective with the following phrase, "We know that we are successful when ... <insert objective here>." This phrase is intended to precede a statement of being or a description of a condition. In other words, objectives should describe the intended outcome in terms of the specific target of the activity; measurable indicators of accomplishment; assignments of responsibility; realistic expectations; and time-bound results [41]. Table 8.1 exemplifies using a prefacing phrase to write objectives in the appropriate tense of the English language. The objective statement's tense is essential as we consider the relationship of objectives and associated activities in the plan. Objectives describe the intended result while activities describe the intermediate actions that achieve that result. Alternately, activities are descriptions of action and begin with a verb (e.g., "Assess water quality," "Distribute water storage containers"). Objectives are descriptions of an entirely successful endpoint and begin with a subject noun that is then modified in the sentence predicate using the passive tense (e.g., "Blankets are distributed," "Children are immunized"). In effect, objectives are measures of effectiveness. This specific sentence structure allows for each of the plan's components to become relational as searchable and sortable data points within the plan database.

Table 8.1. Prefacing phrase used for creating SMART plan objectives

Prefacing phrase	Example of a SMART objective
"We will know that we are successful when ..."	The water department (A) ensures that all (M) people have equal access to 15 liters (M) of safe (R) water (S) per person (M) per day (T).

8.7 Questions for Discussion

1. Describe how objective-based planning offers a means for reducing the uncertainty inherent in emergency operations.

2. Compare execution of an emergency response to performing a play without a script.

   a. Is it possible to perform correctly on opening night?

      i. Is it likely? Why or why not?

   b. How does the likelihood of success change with one person as compared to a group?

   c. Discuss how knowing the ending of the play (i.e., the goal) affects the likelihood of success.

3. Discuss the importance of detail when creating SMART objectives in terms of quantifiable metrics.

Chapter

Capability-Based Planning

9.1 Learning Objectives

Upon completion of the chapter, the reader can:

1. Define the following terms and phrases:
   - Ability
   - Capability inventory
   - Capability-based planning
   - Contingency
   - Critical success factors
   - Function
   - Functional analysis
   - Gap analysis
   - Horizontal management
   - Resource allocation
   - Scenario
   - Scenario-based planning
   - Vertical management.
2. List seven domains of strategic planning described by the mnemonic, "I SIESTA."
   - For each domain, describe the approach and factors that they describe.
3. List three dimensions that influence the capability of a system.
4. Compare critical success factors with measures of success in terms of capability and strategy.
5. List the four steps of capability-based approaches to planning.
6. Recognize the strengths of capability-based planning.

9.2 Approaches to Strategic Planning

Capability-based planning is one of the multiple approaches to strategic planning. Approaches are selected according to the specific requirements and needs of the system intended to serve. "I SIESTA" is the mnemonic used here to recall the approaches for strategic planning. Table 9.1 includes a list and description of these approaches and techniques.

All the techniques are applied as a standardized form of situation analysis intended to describe the current state of affairs related to strategy, quality, influencing factors, and the

Table 9.1. Approaches and techniques for strategic planning [22, 56, 59–63]

Domain	Approach or Technique	Used to describe
Impacts	Effectiveness research	Outcomes
Strategy	SWOT analysis	Strategic position
Influences	Environmental scan	Political, socio-economic, and technological factors
Evidence	Empirical analysis	Quality and quantity
Situation	Scenario-based	Operational and environmental constraints
Threats	Threat-based	Adversaries
Ability	Capability-based	Functionality

system's impacts. The first four entities listed in Table 9.1 represent techniques used to inform strategic planning. These techniques are usually applied early during the data collection phase of the planning process. The final three domains represent approaches that perform strategic planning (e.g., threats, **scenarios**, or capability).

Threats are a dangerous phenomenon, substance, human activity, or condition used to *intentionally* cause loss of life, injury or other health impacts, property damage, loss of livelihoods and services, social and economic disruption, or environmental damage [15]. According to this definition, threats differ from hazards only by human intent. As compared to hazards, threats (and their associated assessments) also include characteristics of the adversary (e.g., intent, prior history, technological ability).

The threat-based approach involves identifying potential adversaries, evaluating their capabilities, and predicting their potential impact. Capability or system requirements are then based on the criterion of outperforming the opposition. Quantitative and qualitative solutions are explored. This threat-based planning approach was common during the Cold War (when adversarial capabilities were relatively well understood) [54].

Scenario-based approaches identify potential hazards, evaluate their likelihood, and predict their potential impacts. System requirements are then based upon the criterion of mitigating losses. This approach utilizes a representative set of situations that are specified in terms of environmental and operational constraints. These scenarios form the testbed for assessing capability or system requirements [54]. Both threat-based and scenario-based planning have a relatively narrow operational focus as compared to capability-based planning.

This narrow focus is no longer practicable for the organizational agility required under dynamic, unpredictable environments [58]. Threat and **scenario-based planning** may imply a degree of false certainty regarding the disaster hazard or threat that is, in fact, unattainable. In addition to limiting the range of solutions, objective-based planning often generates a list without establishing priorities [52]. It is necessary to include a planning approach that addresses this degree of uncertainty regarding our ability to predict disaster risk.

In comparison, capability-based approaches identify the capabilities needed to respond to a broad range of contingencies. **Capability-based planning** allows for more flexible plans to be developed that address a myriad of unpredictable contingencies. This method involves a functional analysis of expected future operations. The result is a description of the functional ability to perform the task to accomplish the objective. A capability inventory is then defined, and the most cost-effective and efficient options to implement these capabilities are derived [54].

9.3 Capabilities

Capabilities describe the functional **ability** to complete activities and achieve desired outcomes (without necessarily specifying the resources involved). The use of capability as a primary currency supports a functional approach to the accomplishment of general requirements [58].

Capabilities have been described as having three dimensions as follows: people, processes, and materials. The people dimension influencing a system's capability includes individual and collective training and professional development. The process dimension of a capability involves its concepts, activities, and management. Finally, the material dimension of capability includes infrastructure, technology, and equipment [59].

A capability takes an extended time to deliver and involves multiple stakeholders producing numerous increments. Therefore, it is useful to divide the capability into strategic goals and operational objectives that deliver discrete, visible, and quantifiable outcomes and outputs from numerous inter-dependent responders. Therefore, strategic goals are also referred to as **critical success factors** in support of the capability. Accordingly, the successful accomplishment of an operational objective represents a "measure of success" supporting the strategic goal. Capabilities provide the common framework used for relating and comparing disparate elements of an emergency response organization.

9.4 Capability-Based Planning

Populations at risk for disasters may face many vastly different hazards and threats within a nearly infinite set of unpredictable scenarios. This unpredictability is best met by planning to accomplish those objectives within our *ability to achieve* (i.e., capability) [13]. Capability-based planning holds substantial advantages over the more traditional threat- and scenario-based planning.

Capability-based planning involves a **functional analysis** of critical operational requirements according to scenarios [60]. Capabilities are identified based on needs. Capability development approaches typically include the following four steps: (1) identify (i.e., inventory) capabilities; (2) assess the level of change required for each capability (i.e., **gap analysis**); (3) prioritize the change required; and (4) develop a plan for implementing change.

Once the required **capability inventory** is defined, the most cost-effective and efficient options to satisfy the requirements are sought [55]. Since it is impossible to predict every given scenario (i.e., terrorists flying airliners into the World Trade Center on September 11, 2001), capability-based planning involves, "Planning under uncertainty to provide capabilities suitable for a wide range of modern-day challenges and circumstances while working within an economic framework that necessitates choice" [55].

The approach of capability-based planning is considered mature. The capability-based approach to planning was initially proposed by Nobel Prize-winning economist Amartya Sen and Martha Nussbaum [64]. The United Nations and development agencies currently assess societies' development using a capability-based approach to create a Human Development Index [61]. Murphy and Gardoni have also proposed using a capability-based approach to measure hazard impact and direct risk analysis and hazard mitigation efforts [13, 62]. At least five nations (i.e., the US, the UK, Australia, Canada, and New Zealand) now use this approach for defense planning [58]. Capability-based planning is also the foundation for which the US Homeland Security Exercise Evaluation Program (HSEEP) and other federal preparedness initiatives are based [13, 22].

The goals of designing the capability-based planning process should include the following determinations [55]:

- whom does what work,
- who has responsibility for the outcome,
- the resources required,
- how long a planning cycle lasts,
- the outcome or outcomes of the process,
- the products to be produced, and
- how the process meets constraints such as timeliness.

9.5 Strengths of Capability-Based Planning

Besides the ability to hedge against a broad range of **contingencies**, capability-based planning also has other characteristics that support its effectiveness. Following is a list of strengths of capability-based planning:

- Facilitates **horizontal management** of capabilities across multiple functions as well as **vertical management** among individual functions [59].
- Provides for cascading of goals from the strategic level down to more detailed operational level objectives and actions.
- Focuses on **function** – "what needs to be done."
- Provides a map of the system's overall capabilities.
- Connects individual capabilities (e.g., knowledge, skills, and abilities, KSAs) with system capabilities.
- Adds priority to objective-based planning.
- Focuses on alternatives and leaves **resource allocation** to the incident manager.
- Provides a systematic way to change major initiatives.

9.6 Questions for Discussion

1. Compare and contrast scenario-based approaches to strategic planning.
2. Compare and contrast scenario-based planning to capability-based planning.
3. Discuss the use of capability-based planning against asymmetrical warfare.

Chapter

10

Consensus-Based Planning

10.1 Learning Objectives

Upon completion of the chapter, the reader can:

1. Define the following terms and phrases:

   - Brainstorming
   - Nominal technique
   - Dialectical inquiry
   - Consensus
   - Voting
   - Delphi method.

2. Recognize Vroom's five processes for decision-making.
3. Compare the following approaches to group decision-making in terms of intentions, attributability, privacy, and majority-rule.
4. List the seven aims of consensus-based planning referred to by the mnemonic, "SPECIES."

10.2 Group Decision-Making

Under normal circumstances, **group decision-making** is considered superior to individualized choices because it not only better informs the process of decision-making with a larger sample of data input, but it also encourages stakeholder creativity, agreement, and accountability. The capacity, depth, and breadth of **knowledge, skills, and abilities** (KSAs) that the group contributes far exceed the value that any individual could contribute to plan-writing.

However, in the case of disaster situations, this form of decision-making is often too slow to keep up with the pace of emergency operations. Instead, incident command systems are designed to facilitate hierarchical control and decision-making. Therefore, the US Federal Emergency Management Agency (FEMA) recommends a group-based approach to writing emergency operations plans (EOPs) [2]. Consensus-based planning allows for deliberative group negotiations to be completed before the crisis occurs. The results of these group negotiations are then documented in the EOP. Thus, the EOP becomes a form of a social contract to be recognized and implemented by the incident commander.

Vroom's normative decision-making model calls for different decision-making methods to be selected according to the specific need [63]. (By the way, how cool is the name, "Vroom"?)

Table 10.1 describes Vroom's five different decision-making processes [63].

A facilitator is an individual who collaborates with a group to facilitate the group's decision-making. The fundamental role of the facilitator is to be a neutral broker of the plan. This role thus excludes them from taking a position in the discussion. Facilitators are typically used to assist groups during consensus-based planning.

10.3 Approaches to Group Decision-Making

Consensus is a form of group decision-making (i.e., collaborative decision-making). Group decision-making occurs when individuals collectively make a choice that is no longer attributable to any single individual. Group decision-making recognizes this social influence on the process.

Table 10.2 compares several major approaches to group decision-making.

All six of the approaches listed in Table 10.2 expectedly involve public group discussion. The distinctions are primarily related to the following factors: (1) intended process and outcome; (2) attributability of alternatives; (3) voting privacy; and (4) majority rule. Each approach is selected according to its specific distinctions.

First off, the intended outcome of these approaches may differ. Brainstorming and the nominal technique seek to generate alternative courses of action, whereas the rest involves a debate of these proposed alternatives. Approaches also differ according to the outcome – resulting

Table 10.1. Vroom's five processes for decision-making

Decision-making process	Description
Decide	Leader makes decision, without consultation or justification.
Consult individuals	Leader consults with individuals. Leader makes decision.
Consults the group	Leader consults entire group. Leader makes decision.
Facilitate	Leader collaborates. Group makes decision.
Delegate	Leader delegates. Group makes decision.

Table 10.2. Examples of major approaches to group decision-making

Approach	Description
Brainstorming	Group publicly generates attributed alternatives, without a decision.
Nominal technique	Group publicly generates non-attributed alternatives, without a decision.
Dialectical inquiry	Group publicly debates non-attributed alternatives, without a decision.
Consensus	Group publicly debates attributed alternatives with a majority decision that is supported by the minority and based upon public agreement.
Voting	Group publicly debates attributed alternatives with a majority decision and based upon private vote.
Delphi	Group publicly debates attributed alternatives with a majority decision and based upon multiple, structured private votes.

in either a final decision or a refined list of possible actions. The first three approaches listed in Table 10.2 (brainstorming, nominal group technique, and dialectical inquiry) represent discussion techniques. While these techniques offer a means for generating and discussing potential courses of action, implicit decision-making still relies upon majority decision through some vote, consensus, or use of the Delphi method.

The second major distinction among these various approaches to group decision-making involves attributing the proposed alternative course of action. The nominal group technique and the dialectical inquiry method intentionally blind the participants regarding the participants' identity that proposed each course of action. This lack of attribution for proposed courses of action is intended to encourage otherwise reticent participants to suggest alternatives with the less perceived social risk from hearing judgment or criticism and reduce individual personalities' effect on the group. Third, approaches differ regarding their use of voting privacy. While all approaches employ the public debates of alternative courses of action, voting and the Delphi method use a private means for voting compared to the public agreement achieved through consensus-based planning. A fourth related distinction involves the use of majority rule versus consensus-based decision-making. Voting and the Delphi method both apply majority rule without revision of that course of action by the dissenting minority. In contrast, consensus-based planning includes a means for additional negotiation and compromise in the decision-making process that then results in consensus among all stakeholders. Buy-in of all stakeholders is thus assured by maintaining a "partnership of equals" (as opposed to the binary "winners and losers" outcome of a voting process).

Consensus and unanimous are not synonymous

10.4 Consensus-Based Decision-Making

In the simplest terms, the definition of consensus is an agreement made by a group. However, this definition does not distinguish consensus-based decision-making from other forms of group decision-making. Consensus-based planning has roots in US Quaker religious communities where the overarching goal was unity rather than unanimity. In the United States, Homeland Security Presidential Directive #8 charged all federal agencies involved in emergency response to participate in emergency planning on a "consensus-basis" [8].

Consensus-based decision-making seeks the agreement of most participants and resolves or mitigates the minority's objections to achieve the most agreeable decision. As mentioned, consensus-based decision-making involves public debate of attributable alternatives followed by a majority decision supported by the minority and based upon the public agreement. The primary requirement of consensus is acceptance by all. If the minority opposes the course of action, it is modified to remove objectionable features and achieve consensus.

Consensus-based decisions are more complicated and time-consuming to reach than a democratic vote or an autocratic decision. Most issues involve trade-offs, and the various decision alternatives will not entirely satisfy everyone. Complete **unanimity** is not the goal – that is rarely possible. However, everyone can have the opportunity to express their opinion, be listened to, and accept a group decision that best aligns with their individual and

Table 10.3. Aims of consensus-based planning

Aim	Description
Supportive	All stakeholders seek the best possible decision for the group
Participatory	All stakeholders actively participate
Egalitarian	All stakeholders have equity of input
Collaborative	All stakeholders contribute to shared proposals and shape them into decisions
Inclusive	All stakeholders are included
Efficient	All stakeholders are respectful of time and scale their input accordingly
Solution-oriented	All stakeholders are expected to compromise to reach a final solution

organizational goals [28]. Neither is consensus **majority rule**. Consensus gives a voice to dissenting opinion and then integrates this perspective into the goals of the group. A consensus decision represents a reasonable decision that all members of the group can accept. It is not necessarily the optimal decision for each member.

The aims of consensus-based planning can be easily recalled using the mnemonic, SPECIES. Table 10.3 describes seven aims of consensus-based decision-making according to the mnemonic for (e.g., supportive, participatory, **egalitarian**, collaborative, inclusive, efficient, and solution-oriented) intentions [28].

10.5 Questions for Discussion

1. How does facilitation differ from other types of group decision-making?

   a. Draw comparisons according to the following factors:

      i. Stakeholder input.
      ii. Responsibility for decision.
      iii. Accountability for decision.
      iv. Stakeholder buy-in.

2. What are the implications of a plan based upon public agreement versus one based on private voting?
3. What characteristic did the Quakers value about consensus-based decision-making?
4. Describe the importance of a "partnership of equals" in terms of consensus.

Compliance with Norms, Plans, and Regulations

11.1 Learning Objectives

Upon completion of the chapter, the reader can:

1. Define the following terms and phrases:
   - Community engagement
   - Compliance management.
2. Describe the two levels of compliance in business operations.
3. Compare the respective roles of disaster planners and incident managers for ensuring compliance with external rules, regulations, and guidelines.
4. Describe the "paper plan syndrome."

11.2 Compliance

For a plan to be effective, stakeholders must first agree to a code of compliance that documents their commitment as a contributor to the mutual goal.

Compliance is the state of following established guidelines or specifications.

The term describes the ability to act according to an order, set of rules, or requests. Compliance is a disaster concern, partly because of an ever-increasing number of guidelines and regulations requiring organizations to understand their specifications fully.

For business operations in general, compliance operates at two levels: (1) compliance with external rules, regulations, guidance and (2) compliance with internal system controls. It is the responsibility of disaster planners to ensure that the plans created are compliant with internal organizational control systems and local, provincial/state, national, and international standards, agreements, and regulations. During emergency operations, this responsibility for ensuring compliance is then transferred to the incident manager, which is delegated to all workers.

11.3 Compliance Management

Compliance management is how managers plan, communicate, organize, control, and lead activities that ensure compliance with laws and standards. These activities can include audits, security procedures, inventory control, reports, and documentation.

In most cases, compliance with the emergency operations plan (EOP) is implied during the group plan-writing process and formally recognized by the signing of the EOP by the stakeholder organization's chief executive before emergency activation. During emergency operations, compliance management is ensured by the incident manager and implemented by the administration and operations chiefs of the incident management system.

Compliance occurs at many levels for emergency operations planning. Firstly, planners are responsible for becoming compliant with internal or external regulations that require a disaster plan to be written in most cases. In many cases, the action of plan-writing itself is a first step in complying with an organizations' risk reduction or emergency preparedness policy.

Unfortunately, this may also be the first opportunity for a common pitfall – "the compliance plan."

As mentioned in Chapter 5, my Coast Guard colleague, Dr. Paul, referred to plans that people write simply to be compliant with writing a plan. Little effort is given to the quality of the plan or effectiveness of its outcomes. The primary aim is to complete the task ("check the box," so to speak) and then move on. My good friend and CDC colleague, Erik Auf der Heide, has also pointed out that the development of poor quality, low impact plans represent a "paper plan syndrome" that may lend a false sense of safety and reassurance because it implies on paper systems that do not function in real life [14].

> "Disaster plans are an illusion unless based upon valid assumptions about human behavior"
>
> – Erik Auf der Heide

In addition to developing and implementing policies and procedures to ensure compliance in disaster planning, we must also develop and implement policies and procedures for disaster planning that ensure compliance. Many of the elements previously described as characteristic of O2C3 planning (e.g., operational-level objectives and capability-based planning built upon consensus) also help promote compliance.

11.4 Compliance with Local Norms

Recent studies of community-based planning in communities at risk for hurricanes have suggested that the most usable interventions are those that engender a high degree of community satisfaction with the engagement process and the intervention content [27].

The challenge is to tailor the disaster planning process to best address various factors, including a community's demographics, location, infrastructure, resources, authorities, and decision-making processes [64]. For this to occur, the respective roles and responsibilities of individuals, families, governments, non-governmental organizations, and the private sector must be based upon social, cultural, economic, environmental, and behavioral norms of the affected population. **Community engagement** is a process for eliciting and integrating these norms into effective operations.

> "Base disaster plans on what people are *likely* to do, not what they *should* do"
>
> – Erik Auf der Heide

Besides social norms, local state and national regulations may also relate to emergency operations. These policies and regulations include the recognition of jurisdictional authority as well as fiscal responsibility. They may also include emergency plans, guidelines, and contingencies developed by the municipal, state/provincial, or national government. These instruments typically represent an attempt at standardized operations and interorganizational coordination with other sectors and jurisdictions.

In addition to these local interorganizational models, compliance with national systems (e.g., the US National Preparedness Goal, the UK Gold-Silver-Bronze command structure, the Australian Health Management Plan for Pandemic Influenza) also provides for a well-established system of controls that may be used to guide local action. National systems offer a hierarchy of plans that connect local needs with national resources.

In addition to local, state/provincial, and national guidelines for emergency operations, there are also numerous resources available for compliance with international standards, best practices, and guidelines. National and regional public health agencies (e.g., the US, China, EU, and Africa Centers for Disease Prevention and Control, Public Health England) routinely develop public information and guidance materials related to emergency management or specific hazards (e.g., Pandemic influenza and COVID-19). The Sphere Project publishes an international standard for humanitarian assistance that includes both a humanitarian charter and detailed descriptions of minimum standards (e.g., nutrition, water, shelter) within a context of human rights [65]. The rights and responsibilities of disaster-related healthcare workers are also detailed within the context of internationally binding agreements, including the Geneva Conventions [66].

11.5 Questions for Discussion

1. Brainstorm to list factors that may tempt disaster planners to cut corners and write a "compliance plan"?

   a. What can be done to lessen this temptation for each of these factors?

2. During the COVID-19 pandemic, many community members did not comply with public health plans for mask-wearing. How can the process of community engagement in disaster planning be used to improve compliance with public policy?

12

The ADEPT™ Planning System

12.1 Learning Objectives

Upon completion of the chapter, the reader can:

1. Define the following terms and phrases:

   - Application
   - Computing platform
   - Dashboard
   - Data
   - Database
   - Database management system
   - Datapoint
   - Hierarchical format
   - Hyperlink
   - Machine learning
   - Quality
   - Quality control
   - Repeatable
   - Reproducible
   - Software
   - Variability

12.2 Introduction to the ADEPT™ Planning System

This chapter describes the ADEPT™ planning system [13, 25–28, 51, 52]. This innovative approach combines the six principles of effective planning (i.e., "O2C3") with a standardized way of storing and retrieving plan information represented by the acronym "SOARR™." The result is an effective and efficient electronic database management **application** that is searchable, sortable, and measurable (compared to an outdated "paper plan" in narrative format).

Electronic **databases** are collections of facts and statistics compiled for reference or analysis (i.e., **data**) specially organized for rapid search and retrieval by a computer. Databases are structured to facilitate the storage, retrieval, modification, and deletion of data in conjunction with various data-processing operations. A **database management system** extracts information from the database in response to queries.

The ADEPT™ system includes both the practices and the principles for effective disaster planning. It includes the methods as well as the tools. Disaster planning activities include writing, storing, sharing, executing, monitoring, and evaluating disaster plans. Thus, the utility of ADEPT™ is not limited to ease of plan-writing. A data management system application also allows for additional functionality related to plan-sharing, real-time update, quality control, dashboard representation, and **machine learning**.

"Necessity is the mother of invention." - *Proverb*

12.3 History of the ADEPT™ Planning System

The ADEPT™ planning system was invented out of necessity. While working at the Centers for Disease Control and Prevention (CDC), I had the ambitious task of assisting six Pacific island nations and territories in writing both hospital and public health plans, a total of twelve plans ... all in one summer!

As is often the case, the process began with a simple tool – the concept of using a table instead of lines in the plan. Tables are universally intuitive, regardless of society. Tables are easily recognizable across strategic goals, objectives, and activities as measures of success (consistent with the logical framework approach depicted in Table 1.2). This universal acceptance was beneficial during the facilitation of group discussions related to the plan. The empty boxes of the table (see Figure 18.1) provided a visual prompt regarding the priority, content, and intent of each **datapoint** in the plan. It also provided a visual reminder for participants to stay on topic. As a facilitator, it became easier to say, "Great story. Now, what should we put in the box?"

As the plans became more extensive and more complex, it then became necessary to cross-reference what had grown to become several sets of tables so that users could quickly switch between tables with just a click. Initially, these tables were represented as hyperlinked tables using word processor software (MS Word). This method (e.g., **hyperlinked** tables) was used to write thirteen separate emergency operation plans (six for hospitals and seven for public health) during 2004.

During 2006–2009, when the CDC's attention turned toward pandemic influenza, planning was recognized as a significant pandemic preparedness component. During this second phase, ADEPT™-style planning at the CDC was expanded to include the entire US state of Florida; the Pacific island nation of Palau; as well as multiple nations in southeast Asia that were affected by outbreaks of H5N1 influenza ("bird flu"), Vietnam, Cambodia, Laos, and Thailand. The planning tool was modestly upgraded to utilize commercial spreadsheet software (MS Excel) with hyperlinked sheet tabs. This application was the first time that the ADEPT™ system was used as a relational database management system. Subsequent versions have recreated this same **computing platform** using commercial database software (MS Access and MS.NET).

During 2008–2011, the third phase of ADEPT™ was implemented to create eighty-seven additional plans for national, municipal, and district jurisdictions in the US, China, Kenya, Tanzania, and Uganda [25, 52]. All these versions used commercial spreadsheet software (MS Excel) with hyperlinked sheet tabs. This file included a table of contents hyperlinked to other spreadsheets, with each sheet tab comprising a separate plan capability. Most recently, ADEPT™ was studied in a fourth phase to guide community-based planning in Puerto Rico and the US Virgin Islands as part of a CDC grant after Hurricane Maria [27].

Along with the ADEPT™ software tool, the process of ADEPT™ planning has also improved. The use of a standardized planning approach accomplished planning in less time, with higher quality and using fewer resources than using a non-standardized approach without a database. The use of a training curriculum for local planners and trainers also appeared to improve planning efforts' sustainability. The use of MS Excel™ as the **software** for a relational database was useful for collecting and presenting planning data – during the planning process and emergency response. This chapter describes the ADEPT™ system and the tool for disaster planning.

12.4 The ADEPT™ System

ADEPT™ is an innovative approach to planning comprised of the following three components:

1. A *format* to organize plan information.
2. A *method* to collect and negotiate plan information.
3. A *platform* to deliver plan data.

12.4.1 Plan Format

ADEPT™ uses a standardized format for organizing plan information (i.e., SOARR™). This standardization of plan format allows for [13]:

- Inter-operability of different plans and plan elements.
- Hierarchical organization of plan elements to avoid redundancy or omissions.
- Integration of objective-based and capability-based planning.
- User-friendly plan viewing by subsequent planners and responders.
- Discrete plan elements to be entered, sorted, and searched within a relational database.
- Quality monitoring, evaluation, and control.

ADEPT™ plan information is organized into a **hierarchical format** data schema consisting of a cascading network of planning elements for each capability. These elements include strategic goals, operational objectives, activities, responsible parties, and standard operating procedures. This hierarchical format cascading from each target capability is referred to as the acronym, "S-O-A-R-R" [13]. Chapter 13 describes the SOARR™ format in detail.

12.4.2 Planning Method

A planning method is a logical way to write a plan. It should be **repeatable** (a measure of internal **variability**) and **reproducible** (a measure of external variability). There are two simple steps in this planning method: preparation and plan-writing (see Chapter 18). Plan preparation involves the convening of stakeholders and the collection and assessment of pertinent background data. The second step involves plan-writing as a group. There, stakeholders convene to review, discuss, teach, learn, negotiate, and agree upon a final plan. Group planning occurs in a plenary session and is closely moderated by a facilitator.

12.4.3 Plan Platform

A platform is an environment in which a piece of software is executed. The ADEPT™ platform is the basic hardware (smartphone/computer) and software (operating system) on which software applications can be run. This environment constitutes the foundation upon which multiple supporting applications can be developed.

The ideal ADEPT™ system platform is one that is [13]:

- easy to use and distribute,
- accessible when needed,
- preserves plan data, and
- technologically appropriate for the user.

The ADEPT™ platform is easily supported by a variety of commercial computing applications, according to the user's needs and preferences. In its simplest iteration, paper hard copies are the primary platform for storing and displaying plan data. Responders engaged in highly austere field conditions may need waterproof hard copies, with checklists and tools related to their specific role. This platform may be preferred under rare and unusually austere technological conditions (e.g., chronic power outage, electromagnetic pulse, radio silence, spark hazard avoidance); in very remote locations (e.g., without cellular or satellite coverage); or in the case of under-trained staff (e.g., not familiar with computers).

A computer, an operating system, and a commercial spreadsheet software program serve as the baseline computing platform for the disaster plan in this book. This platform is handy for facilitating the planning workshops when users need easy access and straightforward viewing of the plan hierarchy and ease of movement throughout the plan. Spreadsheets are also commonly used by many technical professions worldwide, and many stakeholders are, therefore, familiar with their operation and functionality.

Finally, the plan platform can also be represented using a span of data management applications ranging from simple, static forms of database software applications to more sophisticated and dynamic cloud-based operational intelligence applications using big data. Applications may also be integrated to deliver a combined online knowledgebase, document management, content integration, and data security.

12.5 Questions for Discussion

1. Discuss the role of a standardized planning format, the method concerning (internal) repeatability, and (external) reproducibility.
2. Discuss the role of a standardized planning format and method concerning interoperability among stakeholders.
3. People often ask to see a "demo of the ADEPT™ software." How would you respond to this request in terms of describing the ADEPT™ platform?

Chapter

13

The SOARR™ Format for Plan Organization

13.1 Learning Objectives

Upon completion of the chapter, the reader can:

1. Define the following terms and phrases:

   - Basic plan
   - Concept of operations
   - Decision tree
   - Functional annex
   - Hierarchy tree
   - Non-relational data
   - Operational objective
   - Qualitative description
   - Quantitative measure
   - Relational data
   - Resources
   - Responsible party
   - Standard
   - Standardize
   - Standards of practice
   - Strategic goal.

2. Provide an example of one strategic goal for the capability of shelter.
3. Provide an example of at least two operational objectives for that strategic goal.
4. Provide an example of at least three of the activities that accomplish each operational objective.
5. Identify who may be expected to have primary responsibility for each activity.
6. Identify what resources may be needed to accomplish each activity (e.g., number of staff, time, equipment, supplies, cost, and essential information).

13.2 The SOARR™ Format for Plan Organization

Plan elements are comprised of both **relational** and **non-relational data**. Non-relational data includes items associated with a Federal Emergency Management Agency (FEMA)-recommended **Basic Plan** – consisting of the following elements [1]:

- Introductory material.
- Purpose of the plan.

- Current situation and planning assumptions.
- **Concept of operations**.
- Organizational diagrams and assignment of responsibilities.
- Administration and logistics.
- Plan development and maintenance.
- Authorities and references.

Though valuable for plan development and maintenance, this information has less functionality during an emergency response, when time is limited. This information is mainly narrative. It is, therefore, not advantageous or necessary to enter or access in a relational format. It is instead presented summarily under a few tabs or headings in the emergency operations plan (EOP) as non-relational data.

Relational data includes those plan elements described within a FEMA-recommended EOP and the **functional annex** [1]. An EOP draws directly from strategic plans to describe agency and program missions and goals, objectives, and activities. According to self-reported capability, the EOP contains a listing of response capabilities necessary to mount an effective response. This information is best organized according to a cascading network of planning elements for each capability. These five elements that accomplish a capability include the following: (1) **strategic goals**; (2) **operational objectives**; (3) activities; (4) **responsible parties;** and (5) **resources** (e.g., time, labor, cost, materials, essential information). These elements are hereafter referred to by the acronym "SOARR™."

Each capability is associated with one or more strategic objectives that reflect the desired state of affairs intended to be achieved. Each strategic goal is then related to one or more operational objectives, which are, in turn, related to activities that accomplish each operational objective.

Each activity is then associated with a responsible party and resources required to accomplish that activity. This hierarchical format cascading from each capability is referred to as the acronym "SOARR™" and is depicted in Figure 13.1.

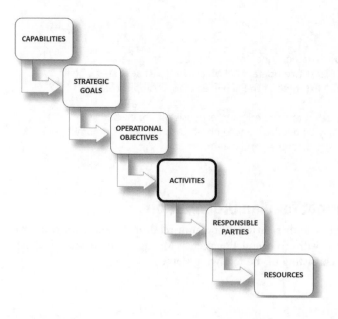

Figure 13.1 Cascade for SOARR™ formatting of EOP relational plan elements.
Source: Adapted from Ciottone 2016 [18]
Permission: Received from Elsevier on December 10, 2020

13.3 Working Definitions

Table 13.1 provides working definitions for this terminology to include general descriptions of capabilities and objectives and definitions for each one of the five elements of SOARR™.

13.4 Hierarchy of Plans

Chapter 1 described an exact organizational format as one of the four characteristics of an effective plan. The ADEPT™ system to planning includes three components: format, method, and platform.

With this planning system, the format of the information is structured according to a standardized hierarchy. Section 1.3 introduced the hierarchy of plans. The ADEPT™ system uses a hierarchy of plans for connecting strategy to action.

Hierarchical plans include strategic, operational, and tactical components that integrate top-level strategic decision-making with lower-level tactical processes (connected by middle-level operations management). The ADEPT™ system uses a planning hierarchy of strategic goals, operational objectives, activities, and tactical resources. For every strategic goal of the plan, there is a set of corresponding operational objectives that accomplish that goal. In turn, there is also a set of activities that accomplish the operational objective. And for each activity, there is an assigned responsible party. Finally, besides primary responsibility for completing the activity, other resources requirements of the activity are identified (e.g., time, labor, cost, materials, and information).

Table 13.1. Working definitions for plan elements

Planning element	Working definition	Simple description
Capability	Ability to achieve a desired operational effect under specified standards and conditions through combinations of means and ways to perform a set of tasks.	Ability
Objectives	A projected state of affairs which a person or a system plans or intends to achieve.	Aim
Strategic goal	A general statement of the intended purpose or intended outcome. Also known as *critical success factors*.	Why
Operational objective	Specific aims that constitute the means for attaining strategic goals. Also known as *measures of success*.	What
Activity	A set of actions that accomplish specific operational objectives. Also known as *tasks*.	How
Responsible parties	Individuals or groups that are assigned responsibility for accomplishing an activity. Responsibility is specified as either primary or secondary.	Who
Resources	A contributing factor that is required to accomplish an activity and achieve a desired outcome. Examples include labor, capital, materials, energy, information, management, and time.	With

Based upon Ciottone 2016 [18]. (Permission received from Elsevier December 10, 2020).

As such, the ADEPT™ system allows for some degree of compartmentalization and specialization for each of the respective stakeholders in the hierarchy (e.g., leader, manager, and worker) while still closely integrating and coordinating the actions of the individual, organizational levels.

13.5 Hierarchy of Hypotheses

Chapter 2 lists FEMA's fourteen principles for developing an all-hazards plan [1]. Those fourteen principles notably include the following three characteristics:

- Plans must identify the mission and supporting goals (with desired results).
- Planning identifies tasks, allocates resources to accomplish those tasks, and establishes accountability.
- Effective plans tell those with operational responsibilities what to do and why to do it. They also instruct those outside the jurisdiction in how to provide support and what to expect.

These three characteristics are effectively addressed by using a method called the hierarchy of hypotheses. The hierarchy of hypotheses is an approach for connecting evidence to theory. The basic tenet behind the hierarchy-of-hypotheses approach is that complexity can often be mastered by hierarchically structuring the topic under study [67].

When separate groups perform planning, the variability among various versions becomes more likely, and it becomes more difficult to reconcile these plans into one information system.

Different plans, all addressing a joint capability or strategic goal, may each address different versions of it, making it hard to reconcile their results. The hierarchy of hypothesis method addresses this challenge by dividing the main hypotheses (or, in our case, strategic goals) into more specific sub-hypotheses (operational objectives) [67]. These hypotheses can be further sub-divided (e.g., measurable activities and resources) until the refinement level allows for direct empirical testing (through simulation, exercise, and actual implementation during real-world disasters).

Thus, in addition to the previously mentioned hierarchy of plans, the ADEPT™ hierarchical format also applies a hierarchy of hypotheses. The result is a tree that visually depicts different ways in which a major hypothesis can be formulated. Decision trees can also be used as support tools for calculating modeling decisions according to their probability, costs, and utility.

The objectives can then be explicitly linked to the tree branch they intend to address, making a conceptual and visual connection to the primary goal. The hierarchical cascade of Figure 13.1 allows us to more intuitively structure and display relationships between different versions of an idea and to conceptually collate actions (or empirical tests) addressing the same overall objectives through divergent approaches.

Figure 13.2 depicts the **hierarchical tree** of the ADEPT™ planning system – consisting of a "trunk" of capability. Emanating from this trunk of capability are the branches of strategic goals that further divide into small branches of operational objectives that terminate in twigs of activity. Finally, each twig of activity is fed by the leaves of resources (e.g., time, labor, cost, equipment, and supplies, information) and staffing.

Table 13.2 represents the same hierarchy as that of Figure 13.2 in a horizontal table format. Planning *ALWAYS* occurs from left to right.

Table 13.2. Hierarchy tree of the APEPT planning approach in table format

Strategic goal 1.0	Operational objective 1.1	Activity 1.1.1	Responsible party A	Human resources Materials Finances Time
		Activity 1.1.2	Responsible party B	Human resources Materials Finances Time
	Operational objective 1.2	Activity 1.2.1	Responsible party C	Human resources Materials Finances Time
		Activity 1.2.2	Responsible party D	Human resources Materials Finances Time

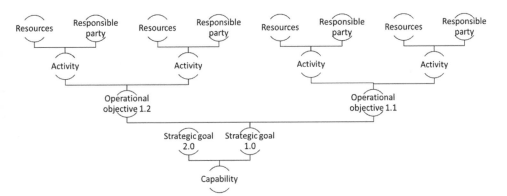

Figure 13.2 Hierarchy tree of the APEPT planning approach

13.6 Integration with the Continuous Quality Improvement Cycle

Figure 13.3 depicts how the ADEPT™ planning cascade (i.e., the SOARR™ format) integrates with the iterative cycles of process improvement (in this case, the Deming cycle) at the level of the plan activity (i.e., process). Chapter 22 discusses how this same

SOARR™ format is used to integrate with the Six Sigma™, another well-known system for process improvement.

13.7 Case Study: Using Sphere Humanitarian Standards in the SOARR™ Planning Format

A **standard** is a measurable norm for the acceptability of quality. **Standards of practice** represent measurable norms for acceptable quality related to performance.

The SOARR™ planning format is easily integrated with a variety of **standardized** resources for emergency response, including the Sphere Project Humanitarian Charter and Minimum Standards for Humanitarian Response [65].

Table 13.3 depicts the close alignment of the corresponding organizational structures for SOARR™ [13] and Sphere formats [65]

Table 13.4 represents an example of how the SOARR™ format is used to depict the hierarchy of plan elements for the Sphere Project standard of "Water, Sanitation, and Hygiene." This example is based upon the Sphere international standards for humanitarian assistance [65]. Appendix B includes an entire sample EOP using Sphere Project standards as the content.

Table 13.3. Corresponding components of the SOARR™ and Sphere information formats

SOARR™	Capability	Strategic objective	Operational objective	Activity	Responsible party	Resources
Sphere	Life-saving activities	Minimum standards	Key indicators	Key actions	Not applicable	Appendices

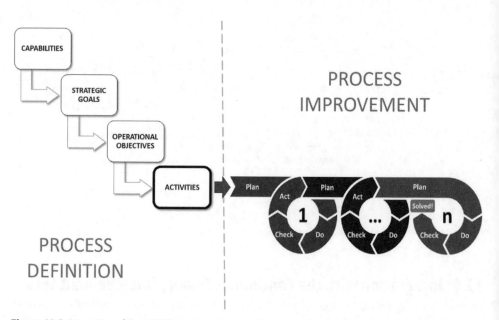

Figure 13.3 Integration of the ADEPT planning cascade with the Deming cycle for continuous quality improvement

Table 13.4 Example of the SOARR™ planning format using Sphere humanitarian standards for water, sanitation, and hygiene

Capability	Strategic Objective	Operational Objective	Activity	Responsible Party	Resources
Water, Sanitation and Hygiene	An adequate supply of clean water is accessible to all people	A sufficient quantity of water is available to all people	Ensure that the maximum distance from any household to the nearest water point is 500 meters Ensure that the average water use for drinking, cooking, and personal hygiene in any household is at least fifteen liters per person per day	Public works	Staffing Time Equipment Transportation Communications
		Water is of sufficient quality to be potable and used for hygiene	Ensure there is low risk of fecal contamination Use a sanitary survey to indicate the risk of fecal contamination Ensure there are no fecal coliforms per 100 milliliters at the point of delivery	Sanitarian	Staffing Time Testing equipment Survey tool Transportation Communications
		People are able to safely collect, store, and use sufficient quantities of water	Ensure each household has at least two clean water collecting containers of ten-to-twenty liters Ensure water collection and storage containers have narrow necks and/or covers (or other safe means of storage, drawing, and handling)	Central supply	Staffing Time Containers Transportation Communications

Source: Based upon Ciottone, 2016 [18]
Permission: Received from Elsevier December 10, 2020 and from Sphere Project January 4, 2021

13.8 Phrasing of Plan Content for the SOARR™ Format

Using a standardized plan hierarchy requires standardized phrasing for plan elements (i.e., capabilities, goals, objectives, activities, responsible parties, and resources). Plan elements must also be phrased according to their intended use as operational instructions for the end-user. Capabilities, responsible parties, and resources are written using descriptive terms, usually as one or a brief phrase. In contrast, goals, objectives, and activities are written in quantitative terms and should *ALWAYS* be written as a *complete* sentence. It is essential to write complete and free-standing sentences since the plan's elements are stored separately in a database that may be searched and sorted independent of other plan statements. Full sentences stand alone when read, regardless of their context or placement within the plan. Complete sentences are also an essential aim for stakeholders when writing the plan together. Complete sentences capture a greater deliberation level than required to utter a one- or two-word phrase (e.g., when brainstorming). Full sentences include both a subject and an object. The best complete sentences for planning include precise nouns and verbs in a simple subject-predicate format.

Besides using complete sentences, the tense of the sentence is also important. For goals and objectives, we use the present tense and passive voice. These sentences typically include a subject noun, a nonaction verb, and then a predicate noun or modifier. For example, the strategic goal is that "Sufficient water is available to everyone." The operational goal is that "All persons received fifteen liters of water per day."

Goals and objectives are written to describe what a successful outcome looks like *after it has been accomplished*. For example, the plan should state that "Water *is* available," not "Water *will be* available."

For that reason, I often remind stakeholders to (silently) preface their ideas for goals and objectives with the phrase, "We know we're successful when ... <insert phrasing here>." This prefacing helps us to state the passive voice and to plan in measurable terms.

It is also important to note that the strategic goal is written as a **qualitative description** of the intended outcome (e.g., "Sufficient water is available to everyone"). In contrast, the operational objective is written as a **quantitative measure** of a successful outcome (e.g., "All persons receive fifteen liters of water per day").

In contrast to goals and objectives, activities are stated in the present tense as commands in the active voice. These sentences typically begin with an action verb and end with a noun or modifier (e.g., "Deliver the water daily").

13.9 Questions for Discussion

1. Compare and contrast the hierarchy of plans with the hierarchy of hypotheses.
2. Describe the role of standardization related to plan nomenclature, plan organizational format, and phrasing of plan content.
3. Draw a hierarchy table for the capability of making breakfast.

Chapter

14

The ADEPT™ Planning Wheel

14.1 Learning Objectives

Upon completion of the chapter, the reader can:

1. Define the following terms and phrases:
   - Affective
   - Assumption
   - Assumption-based planning
   - Cognitive
   - Exercises
   - Functional ability
   - Psychomotor
   - Risk assessment
   - Simulations
   - Situation assessment.
2. List the five phases of the ADEPT™ planning wheel.
3. List the two components of planning assumptions.
4. Compare and contrast implicit and explicit planning assumptions.
5. Describe how functional ability is a strategic measure of quality.
6. Recognize the five essential resources included in a mission area plan.
7. Describe the purpose of the gap analysis.
8. Compare and contrast the creation of a mission area plan with that of a preparedness plan.
9. List six methods used to test communications and operational practices of a plan.

14.2 The ADEPT™ Planning Wheel

Figure 14.1 represents the ADEPT™ planning wheel, a system for creating and evaluating mission area plans. The wheel incudes fifteen steps organized into five phases.

As illustrated in Figure 14.1, the ADEPT™ planning system includes the following five phases that can be recalled by the mnemonic, "AC3T."

1. Assess planning *assumptions*.
2. Create a mission area *plan*.
3. Check the mission area plan for *gaps* related to planning assumptions.

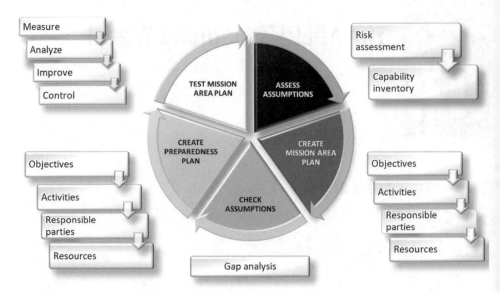

Measure

Analyze

Improve

Control

Risk assessment

Capability inventory

Objectives

Activities

Responsible parties

Resources

Objectives

Activities

Responsible parties

Resources

TEST MISSION AREA PLAN

ASSESS ASSUMPTIONS

CREATE PREPAREDNESS PLAN

CREATE MISSION AREA PLAN

CHECK ASSUMPTIONS

Gap analysis

Figure 14.1 The ADEPT™ (AC3T) planning wheel

4. Create a *preparedness* plan to correct the gaps.
5. Test the plan for the *efficiency* of performance and *effectiveness* of outcomes.

Table 14.1 provides a logical framework for the ADEPT™ planning system, as applied to emergency operations planning for the response mission area.

14.3 Assess Planning Assumptions

In the first phase of the wheel, stakeholders convene to assess assumptions upon which the plan is based. As introduced in Section 2.2, disasters are defined by "losses which exceed the ability of the affected community . . ." **Planning assumptions** explicitly describe needs and resources based upon our best predictions of the future. Planning assumptions are based upon a prediction of future **situations.** These descriptions of needs and resources are often referred to as **situation assessment**.

There are two steps involved in assessing planning assumptions: (1) **risk assessment** – predicting needs and describing the **functional ability** of stakeholders to address those needs and (2) a capability inventory.

Assumption-based planning is one approach to strategic planning developed by RAND to help organizations to deal with uncertainty. It's most often used when future results cannot be easily extrapolated from experience [36]. Section 9.2 introduced the mnemonic, "I SIESTA," used to recall seven strategic planning approaches. Table 9.1 lists and describes these approaches and techniques. Key among these are the approaches related to scenario-based, threat-based, and capability-based planning.

According to Table 9.1, planning assumptions associated with scenario-based and threat-based planning describe the situation's future constraints. Alternately, planning assumptions for capability-based planning describe future functional *ability* [55, 58]. This allows for more flexible plans to be developed that address a myriad of unpredictable contingencies.

Table 14.1. Logical framework for creating an emergency operations plan (EOP)

Planning phase	Focus	Process	Activity	Outputs
Assess assumptions	Hazards	Risk assessment	Hazard identification	Planning assumptions
	Consequences		Hazard characterization	
	Impacts		Impact analysis	
	Risk		Risk characterization	
	Capability	Capability inventory	Capability identification	
			Capability description	
Create EOP	Ability	Capability based planning	Write capabilities	Emergency operations plan
		Objective-based planning	Write objectives (S-O)	
		Operational planning	Write activities (A)	
		Tactical planning	Assign responsibilities (R)	
			Allocate resources (R)	
Check assumptions	Capacity	Gap analysis	Capacity analysis	Gap analysis report
			Capacity comparison	
Create preparedness plan	Ability	Capability-based planning	Write capabilities	Preparedness plan
		Objective-based planning	Write objectives (S-O)	
		Operational planning	Write activities (A)	
		Tactical planning	Assign responsibilities (R)	
			Allocate resources (R)	
Test EOP	Readiness	Process measurement	Process measurement	Process run and control charts
			Quantitative analysis	
		Process control	Process improvement	Corrective action plans
			Process control	

14.4 Create a Mission Area Plan

The second phase of the ADEPT™ planning wheel is to create a plan for one of the five mission areas (i.e., prevention, protection, mitigation, response, and recovery). This book completes a disaster plan for the mission area of response (i.e., an EOP). This process of planning begins with the capabilities identified in the planning assumptions.

Once planning assumptions have been established, a mission area plan is then created based upon the capability and capacity evidenced in those planning assumptions. Stakeholders use the SOARR™ format to describe their mutual intentions for each capability in the plan. Resources may be further specified for each activity in the mission area plan (e.g., responsible parties, staffing, time, cost, materials, and essential elements of information).

Using consensus, stakeholders draft strategic goals and operational objectives that clearly state the expected outcomes related to each capability. Stakeholders then collaborate to identify activities and responsible parties that accomplish these strategic goals and operational objectives using the available capacity (i.e., essential resources, including staffing, funding, materials, time, and information).

14.5 Check the Plan for Gaps Related to Planning Assumptions

The third phase of the planning wheel is gap analysis related to the planning assumptions. The purpose of the gap analysis is to identify gaps between the *predicted* levels of needs and the current *actual* capacity. These gaps between the predicted capacity ($Capacity_{Predicted}$) and the actual capacity ($Capacity_{Current}$) then become the focus of a subsequent preparedness plan intended to build operational capacity to levels that are essential for adequate functionality.

After creating the mission area plan, the next phase is to check (i.e., validate) it against the planning assumptions. This gap analysis compares currently held capabilities and capacity with those predicted by the risk assessment. The gap analysis intends to identify and then quantify any planning assumptions deficiencies before creating a preparedness plan that actively commits resources to build stakeholder capacity.

14.6 Create a Preparedness Plan to Correct the Gaps

The fourth phase of the ADEPT™ planning wheel is creating a preparedness plan that fills these gaps in functional ability. The preparedness plan includes a comprehensive set of objectives, activities, responsible parties, and associated resources that will accomplish any remediation necessary to build adequate capacity among these core capabilities and essential functions.

Any gaps in capability or capacity are prioritized as the objectives for an all-hazard preparedness plan that corrects these gaps within a specific timeframe. The preparedness plan is then implemented according to the preparedness cycle (see Figure 2.1) and typically involves elements related to the "eleven E's of emergency preparedness" (see Table 3.1). The preparedness plan implementation process is actively monitored and evaluated for productivity during and at the end of each operational period (see Table 1.1) The plan should also include monitoring and evaluation components using a validated system for process improvement (see Figure 13.3).

14.7 Test the Mission Area Plan for the Efficiency of Performance and Effectiveness of Outcomes

Finally, the fifth phase of the ADEPT™ planning wheel is to test the plan for the efficiency of performance and effectiveness of outcomes. This testing process usually occurs incrementally, starting with **cognitive** simulations (e.g., gaming, tabletop exercises) and progressing to more complex **psychomotor** and **affective exercises**. Plan activities are monitored and evaluated for efficiency (in terms of resource utilization rates during plan execution) and outcome effectiveness (in terms of accomplishing operational objectives of the plan).

According to the US National Preparedness System, stakeholders should plan for each of the five mission areas (i.e., prevention, protection, mitigation, response, and recovery). In effect, this means that a comprehensive preparedness program should include five separate planning wheels, one for each mission area. While there may be some degree of overlap, in many cases, the capabilities are quite different. For example, capabilities related to land-use zoning and building codes are often included in plans related to the mission area of mitigation, but not for a response.

14.8 Case Study: Welcome to Pyronesia

For this book, we consider the fictitious nation of "Pyronesia" for our case study as we apply the principles of ADEPT™ planning to practice. Throughout the rest of this book, our case study relates to Pyronesia as we assess planning assumptions, create an EOP, check our assumptions through a gap analysis, create a preparedness plan that addresses those gaps, and test our EOP through simulation and, ultimately, using artificial intelligence (see Figure 14.2).

For our case study, Pyronesia is a small, landlocked nation located in a temperate four-season climate. Nearly all this low-resource-country is situated within a large, expansive valley encircled by mountains containing six "Great Lakes" (all located in neighboring nations). The lighter area in the right upper corner is known to be seismically active. The small shaded grey area located in the upper central inland is the capital city, "Caldera." Seventy-five percent of the nation's one million citizens live in the capitol city. The one international airport in the country, Koshiba Field, is also located there. Much of the country (except for the capitol) is linked by a rail system (shown in white). Fifty percent of the roadways are unpaved.

The country is governed as a loosely-affiliated Presidential republic consisting of fourteen (relatively autonomous) provinces – each with a powerful provincial governor. There is a small national military defense force. The economy is chiefly agrarian and dependent upon the fertile inland hills and valleys where many coffee plantations and vineyards are located. Twenty-five percent of the population lives below the poverty line. Fifty percent of the population is over the age of fifty years old.

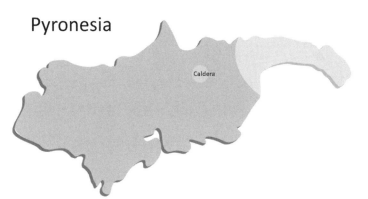

Pyronesia

Caldera

Figure 14.2 The fictitious nation of Pyronesia

14.9 Questions for Discussion

1. Compare and contrast the ADEPT™ planning wheel with Deming's quality control loop and Fayol's five functions of management.
2. Explain why mission area plans are written before preparedness plans.
3. Compare and contrast the three phases of the ADEPT™ planning wheel that perform evaluations with those two phases that create plans.

Preparation for Plan-Writing

15.1 Learning Objectives

Upon completion of the chapter, the reader can:

1. Define the following terms and phrases:
   - Core Planning Team (CPT)
   - Mandate
   - Lead planner (LP)
   - Planning workgroup (PW).
2. Recognize the twelve project objectives for writing an EOP.

15.2 "Planning to Plan"

Planning is a complex task performed by a group of individuals – usually for an essential purpose. It then makes sense to plan such an endeavor. For this reason, the first step in developing an emergency operations plan (EOP) is "planning to plan." In other words, developing a plan for the disaster planning project itself.

We may therefore use the SOARR™ format to organize our plan information. First off, the mission area that we intend to address determines the capabilities needed in our project plan. In this case, we are writing a response plan (i.e., EOP). Strategic goals are then written for each capability. One strategic goal of this project plan could be "A public health EOP is available to guide multi-sectoral emergency response operations, in the event of disaster declaration." Operational objectives are then created to accomplish the strategic goal.

Table 15.1 offers a list of operational objectives (i.e., measures of success) for planning to write an EOP.

Disaster planners should consider these objectives as the basis for writing their project plans for creating an EOP by adding activities and responsible parties to each of the twelve objectives identified in Table 15.1. Following is a discussion of each objective.

15.3 There Is a Clear Mandate to Write an EOP

For planning to occur, there must be a clear mandate to write the EOP. This mandate usually comes as an official order from formal authority. In US hospitals, the Joint

Table 15.1. Twelve project objectives for writing an EOP

1. There is a clear **mandate** to write an EOP.
2. An experienced planner is assigned the responsibility to lead the disaster planning project.
3. A **planning workgroup** (PW) is convened among plan stakeholders.
4. All plan stakeholders understand their own respective roles in the project.
5. All plan stakeholders have the knowledge, skills, and ability to use the ADEPT™ planning system.
6. PW members have collected background data and references related to the EOP (see Section 13.2 and Table 4.4).
7. PW members are reconvened to draft planning assumptions, which include the following:
   a. Risk assessment,
   b. Capability inventory.
8. Lead planner (LP) and Core Planning Team (CPT) have created a draft non-relational Basic Plan (see Section 13.2).
9. PW members are reconvened to review, edit, and agree upon non-relational data in the Basic Plan.
10. All plan stakeholders are convened to draft strategic goals and operational objectives (i.e., "S-O").
11. All plan stakeholders are reconvened to draft EOP activities, assign responsible parties and identify essential resources (i.e., adding "A-R-R").
12. All plan stakeholders are reconvened to authorize the EOP.

Commission for Accreditation of Hospital Organizations (JCAHO) includes the maintenance of a hospital EOP as a requirement for accreditation. Hospital boards and administrations, therefore, commonly mandate the creation and maintenance of an EOP. Among US state, local, tribal, and territorial public health agencies, this mandate is usually associated with funding eligibility (e.g., the CDC Public Health Emergency Preparedness Program, PHEP).

However, in other cases, the mandate may not be so explicit. This lack of a clear mandate is especially challenging when no plan has existed in the past. In these instances, roles and responsibilities are likely to remain unclear. An unclear mandate may also be couched within this uncertainty. For example, as a lead public health planner, I had the opportunity to work with multiple national-level public health agencies to develop their EOPs for the first time. At the time, these EOPS were relatively innovative in that, while they were led by public health, multiple governmental and nongovernmental sectors implemented them. This convening of multiple stakeholders across sectors is not a routine occurrence and implies a certain level of buy-in and perhaps, in some cases, intervening governance. And there have been several occasions when essential stakeholders were absent from the initial convening but then participated in subsequent meetings after a quick telephone reminder from the President!

But to be fair, there is a careful balance of risk and benefit when stakeholders assess the relatively labor-intensive process of disaster planning and weigh their participation level. It is most helpful (and in some cases even necessary) when the chief executive (e.g., President, Prime Minister, CEO, health minister, hospital administrator) issues a formal statement of mandate in advance. This message communicates to all stakeholders the authority of this policy and the importance of active participation. It also speaks to the rewards and benefits of such action.

15.4 An Experienced Planner Is Assigned the Responsibility to Lead the Disaster Planning Project

As with any project, it is essential to assign leadership and to delegate responsibility. There should be a lead planner (LP) assigned to all disaster planning projects. Ideally, the lead planner should be experienced in both preparedness and response. However, a good planner need not have prior disaster experience. It is more important that planners are logical, linear thinkers with an eye for detail and the patience to ensure stakeholdership.

Depending upon the size, the LP is usually supported by several staff members. This **core planning team** (CPT) should also include the workshop facilitator and individuals working to assist the administrative and logistical requirements of subsequent plan writing events (e.g., communications, clerical, audiovisual services, and facilities staff).

15.5 A Planning Workgroup (PW) Is Convened among Plan Stakeholders

The next step in preparing to plan is to identify and convene a multi-sectoral planning workgroup (PW) to manage the disaster planning project itself. The workgroup should comprise five-to-ten individuals able to participate in discussions regarding capabilities to be included in the EOP. PW members should have a general working knowledge of the institution's response capabilities or jurisdiction that they are representing.

15.6 All Plan Stakeholders Understand Their Respective Roles in the Project

Once convened, it is now the LP and CPT's responsibility to develop an orientation that will describe the project to the PW and all stakeholders involved in planning.

Besides their roles and responsibilities as stakeholders (and potential future implementers) of the EOP, all stakeholders must also learn what commitments may be necessary during the disaster planning project itself (e.g., time, subject matter expertise, materials, and management).

15.7 All Plan Stakeholders Have the Knowledge, Skills, and Ability to Use the ADEPT™ Planning System

In addition to their roles and responsibilities during the project, all plan stakeholders also require training to give them the knowledge, skills, and ability to use the ADEPT™ system. At a minimum, all stakeholders involved in writing the EOP should describe the ADEPT™ planning wheel, the SOARR™ table format, the O2C3 approach, and working definitions for the primary plan elements (see Table 13.1). This training may be provided at the same time as the project orientation described in Section 15.5.

15.8 Planning Workgroup Members Collect Background Data and References Related to the EOP

Once familiar with the mission and process, PW members then collaborate to collect background data and references related to the EOP. Table 15.2 lists some of the background data that may be helpful to inform an EOP.

Table 15.2. Examples of background data and references collected to inform an EOP

- Maps (e.g., topography, demography, disaster hazards, critical infrastructure, social vulnerability)
- Emergency plans (e.g., preparedness, response, recovery, contingency)
- Pertinent after-action reports and research related to exercises and real events
- Risk assessments and hazard-vulnerability analyses (HVAs)
- Response handbooks, guides, and references
- Hazard data (type, historical frequency, location, likelihood, impact)
- Population data (demographics, health status, social vulnerability index)
- Hazard-specific guidelines (e.g., hazardous materials operations, pandemic guides)
- Information exchange data (e.g., requirements for essential elements of information, communications, data exchange and information security)
- Contact information for all responsible parties to be named in the EOP

15.9 Planning Workgroup Members Are Reconvened to Draft Planning Assumptions

In this objective, PW members reconvene to draft planning assumptions. As discussed in Chapter 14, these planning assumptions are based upon a risk assessment and a capability inventory. During the risk assessment, disaster hazards are identified and prioritized according to their likelihood and scale of impact. These impacts and their associated health consequences are then evaluated. This hazard characterization identifies the mismatch of needs and resources created by disaster hazards and aligns functional abilities to address those needs (see Tables 4.1–4.3). Finally, the planning assumptions include a capability inventory – listing current core capabilities that apply to the specific emergency needs.

These analytical activities are best performed in a small workgroup setting with the opportunity for frequent discussions and iterations of thought. The entire process begins with a relatively well-defined and scripted process for risk assessment and capability inventory and ends with consensus-based decision-making regarding the group's capabilities. This process is best performed in a live group setting or as a virtual review of a shared document because it requires real-time back-and-forth discussion, not readily amenable to email.

15.10 Lead Planner and Core Planning Team Create a Draft Nonrelational Basic Plan

Once the PW has drafted planning assumptions, the LP (and CPT) may create a draft Basic Plan. As detailed in Section 13.2, plan elements may be considered as essentially comprised of both relational and nonrelational data. Nonrelational data includes items associated with a Federal Emergency Management Agency (FEMA)-recommended "Basic Plan" – consisting of the following elements [1]:

- Introductory material.
- Purpose of the plan.
- Current situation and planning assumptions.
- Concept of operations.
- Organizational diagrams and assignment of responsibilities.
- Administration and logistics.

- Plan development and maintenance.
- Authorities and references.

15.11 Planning Workgroup Members Are Reconvened to Review, Edit, and Agree upon Nonrelational Data in the Basic Plan

Based on the planning assumptions (and subsequent interviews with plan stakeholders and other subject matter experts, as needed), the LP and CPT then draft a Basic Plan, including non-relational data, as described in Section 15.10. These planners then reconvene with the PW to review, edit, and agree upon nonrelational data in a facilitated group session. The final output of this session is the Basic Plan for the EOP.

15.12 All Plan Stakeholders Are Convened to Draft Capabilities, Strategic Goals, and Operational Objectives

Once the PW has completed its work related to the planning assumptions and basic plan, it represents the first time all plan stakeholders are convened to plan together. All plan stakeholders are then convened in a closely facilitated plenary session to review and draft strategic goals and operational objectives for the EOP. This group of stakeholders typically includes twenty-to-fifty active participants.

For expediency, these goals and objectives may also be drafted in advance by the LP and CPT and then presented to all plan stakeholders during the plenary session. This session is then used to review, discuss, learn about, propose, and finalize the strategic goals and operational objectives for the EOP. In other words, the output of this session is a strategic plan for emergency operations.

15.13 All Plan Stakeholders Are Reconvened to Draft EOP Activities, Assign Responsible Parties, and Identify Essential Resources

All plan stakeholders then reconvene for another plenary planning session that drafts activities that accomplish all strategic plan objectives. During the same session, stakeholders also decide those parties responsible and resources that may be essential for accomplishing each activity. However, this session is slightly different than the strategic planning session in that less of these elements may be predicted and drafted in advance by the lead planner and core planning team. In previous studies, approximately fifty percent of the lead planner's activities drafted in advance were changed by stakeholders during the planning session. It should also be noted that even though the stakeholders change these activities, it is useful to have a set of draft activities for consideration. Plan stakeholders do not have to "begin with an empty slate," so to speak.

15.14 All Plan Stakeholders Are Reconvened to Authorize the EOP

In this final session for plan writing, stakeholders convene one last time to review and authorize the EOP as a group. In this setting, all the plan stakeholders commit to the authorship of the plan. This convergence serves a dual purpose in both the practical sense of establishing version control and the aspirational sense of celebrating the accomplishment and partnership.

15.15 Questions for Discussion

1. Describe why it is essential for there to be a clear mandate to write an EOP?
2. It is assumed that effective plans could be written in less time if there are fewer stakeholders involved. Unfortunately, this is not the case. Why so?
3. What role does involvement in plan-writing play in commitment to the intended group outcome?

Chapter

Planning Assumptions

16

16.1 Learning Objectives

Upon completion of the chapter, the reader can:

1. Define the following terms and phrases:
   - Competency-based learning
   - Competent
   - Core competency
   - Microsoft Access™ database
   - Microsoft Excel™ spreadsheet
   - Microsoft SQL Server™ database
   - Microsoft Word™ word processor
   - Server
   - Strategic capability.

2. List the four components of functional ability.
3. List the five phases (i.e., mission areas) included in comprehensive emergency management planning programs.
4. List the five phases of the ADEPT™ planning cycle.
5. Describe the two steps involved in the assessment of planning assumptions.
6. List the four main steps of risk assessment.
7. Describe the goal of a capability inventory.

16.2 Strategic Capability

In Chapter 1, we described the organizational hierarchy of processes, operations, and strategy. Within this context, Table 1.1 defined ability as a measure of quality related to strategic goals. In this sense, ability (i.e., the means to accomplish a goal) is a measurable **strategic capability** indicator.

In this same model, a strategic capability is defined as the ability to accomplish an intended strategic goal. Strategic capability is achieved when outputs and outcomes result in the ability to accomplish a strategic goal.

Standardization of a strategic capability allows managers to plan, organize, staff, direct, and control predictable activities that ensure outcomes with a substantially higher degree of certainty (i.e., validity and reproducibility) and productivity (i.e., effectiveness and efficiency).

16.3 Core Capabilities, Functional Ability, and Competency

Capabilities are considered core if they are critical to the accomplishment of a strategic goal. An organization's core capabilities are evolving at any given point, and strategic capability depends upon successfully managing that evolution.

As introduced in Chapter 9, capabilities have been described as having three dimensions: people, processes, and materials. Core capabilities include material resources (such as facilities, equipment, and supplies) and the processes and human resources to accomplish the process.

All five actions of the preparedness cycle (i.e., organize/equip; train; exercise; evaluate/improve; and plan) are designed to build and maintain core capabilities by applying human and material resources via functional processes (see Figure 2.1). Human resources impart **functional ability**, the means for the successful performance of the activities involved.

Figure 16.1 depicts the relationship between four components of functional ability as follows: (1) employee knowledge and skills applied to; (2) technical systems guided by; (3) managerial systems that are embedded within; and (4) social values and norms [68].

For example, in the case of emergency management, staff knowledge, skills, and abilities regarding water, sanitation, and hygiene are applied to technical systems of environmental health; then directed by emergency managers (within an incident command system); according to local, state, national and international norms (e.g., Sphere Project humanitarian standards).

Core competencies describe standardized levels of employee/worker performance in terms of the knowledge, skills, and abilities (KSAs) needed to accomplish a core capability when given adequate resources. In turn, the staff is deemed **competent** when able to demonstrate the appropriate KSAs. **Competency-based learning** is intended to measure the effectiveness of staff performance and training needs in terms of these KSAs. Thus, the KSAs are a standard model for staff training goals.

16.4 Determining the Mission Area of Emergency Management

As introduced in Chapter 2, comprehensive disaster planning should include plans for all five mission areas of emergency management: prevention, protection, mitigation, response,

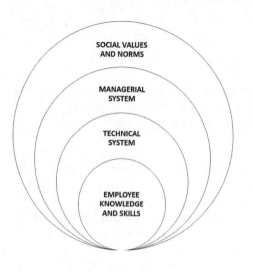

Figure 16.1 Four components of functional ability

SOCIAL VALUES
AND NORMS

MANAGERIAL
SYSTEM

TECHNICAL
SYSTEM

EMPLOYEE
KNOWLEDGE
AND SKILLS

and recovery. Therefore, the first step in determining plan content is determining the mission area of emergency management for which the plan is intended.

Some of the same capabilities apply to multiple mission areas of emergency management. But the stakeholders, processes, and outcomes are relatively unique for other mission areas. For this reason, it is recommended that five separate plans be developed – one for each mission area of emergency management. Accordingly, each of these five plans should also be accompanied by a corresponding preparedness plan that details the activities and objectives of preparing to perform that phase of emergency management.

This book describes the ADEPT™ planning wheel as applied to planning for the response mission area (see Figure 3.2).

However, the same process may also be used for capabilities associated with any of the five mission areas of emergency management (e.g., prevention, protection, mitigation, response, and recovery). Perhaps somewhat counter-intuitively, this five-step planning wheel begins by first writing a plan for the mission area, then writing the corresponding preparedness plan for improving and maintaining capabilities during that phase (using the five-step preparedness cycle) (see Figure 2.1). Thus, the ADEPT™ planning wheel serves as a framework for applying Deming's quality control loop to Fayol's five management functions with the goal of readiness to perform each phase of emergency management.

16.5 Assessing Planning Assumptions

RAND defines an assumption as "an assertion about some characteristic of the future that underlies the current operations or plans of an organization" [36]. Planning assumptions are either implicit or explicit. Explicit assumptions are clearly stated in the plan without ambiguity. Implicit assumptions are not expressed and may go undetected. As such, they may also be a source of uncertainty and affect emergency operations plan (EOP) efficiency or effectiveness. It is, therefore, better to make explicit statements of planning assumptions that accurately guide strategic planning.

Figure 16.2 illustrates the first phase of the ADEPT™ planning wheel – assessment of planning assumptions. The assessment of EOP planning assumptions includes two steps, a risk assessment and a capability inventory for response operations.

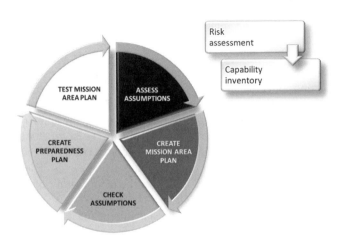

Figure 16.2 Two steps involved in assessment of planning assumptions, as the first phase of the planning wheel

Planning assumptions reflect the expected mismatch of needs and resources (e.g., risk and capability) characteristic of disaster response. According to the definition of disaster in Chapter 2 that describes disasters as a mismatch of needs and resources, disaster response needs are identified by a risk assessment, and a capability inventory identifies resources.

16.6 Risk Assessments

The goal of risk assessment is to quantify the probability of a future outcome along with a statement of uncertainty regarding the assessment itself.

Risk assessments typically include three main steps as follows:

1. Hazard analysis – identification, and description of disaster hazards, likelihood, and consequences,
2. Impact analysis – quantitative description of health consequences, and
3. Risk characterization – integrating the joint probability of hazards and impacts into one risk estimate and statement of uncertainty.

Chapter 17 discusses these four steps of risk assessment in more detail.

16.7 Capability Inventory

Once the risk assessment is performed, capabilities are then self-identified and inventoried by the plan stakeholders. This capability inventory aims to describe the quality and quantity of stakeholder capabilities to address disaster-related needs identified in the risk assessment. Capability inventories typically involve a listing accompanied by descriptions of stakeholder capabilities. Capability assessments are qualitative. They involve the identification and description of the capabilities that stakeholders use to accomplish the plan.

The preparedness gap analysis begins with resource management. A capability inventory is a form of resource typing.

The brainstorming approach described in Table 10.2 is an effective method for initiating the capability inventory. Stakeholders are initially asked to brainstorm and self-identify their respective capabilities to respond to disasters' fifteen most common public health consequences (see Tables 4.1–4.3). A final draft inventory of capabilities is then decided using stakeholder consensus. This capability inventory summarizes the collective core capabilities of the organizational incident command system.

Both the private and public sectors possess many potential mission area capabilities described according to increasing levels of detail. For example, Table 3.3 provides a detailed listing of core capabilities of "ESF #8 – Public Health and Medical Services." These capabilities reflect the actions of the public health and medical sector, regardless of the specific disaster hazard. These listings offer various selections for public health emergency planners to consider as they identify content for their plan (see Table 4.3).

Using this capability-based approach, stakeholders can respond to disasters by applying their inherent capabilities to all disaster risks, regardless of hazard priority. These capability inventories also form a baseline for measuring and tracking response capabilities that may be further validated by data derived from exercises, simulations, and actual events. These resultant capabilities represent the foundation of an EOP and form the main "trunk" of the EOP hierarchical decision tree (see Figure 13.2).

Once this capability inventory is defined, an EOP is developed that implements the most cost-effective and efficient options for achieving functional ability among all capabilities

[54]. Thus, as initially introduced in Table 1.1, functional ability is a measure of quality applied to capability.

16.8 Case Study: Planning Assumptions for Pandemic Influenza Response in Southeast Asia

16.8.1 Background

In 2004, a major new outbreak of highly pathogenic H5N1 influenza (i.e., avian influenza or "bird flu") surfaced in Vietnam and Thailand's poultry industry, and within weeks spread to ten countries and regions in Asia (with limited human transmission). In 2005, the US developed a national strategy for pandemic influenza, and by 2007 the Centers for Disease Control and Prevention (CDC) deployed several hundred personnel (including this author) to work in pandemic preparedness throughout Asia should the virus mutate to become transmissible.

In 2008, I was asked to lead CDC's regional pandemic influenza planning efforts in Vietnam, Thailand, Laos, and Cambodia. Our objective was to assist these nations in developing and implementing a multi-sectoral, consensus-based planning model at the provincial level. Once the plans were in place, these nations would also become eligible for additional assistance from the World Health Organization (WHO), including access to a regional stockpile of public health and medical materials. In this case, it would be necessary to develop pandemic plans de novo, where none had existed before. The challenge of deciding appropriate plan content was formidable, not only because pandemic planning was a new precedent for these nations. The challenge also related to the economic and political differences spanning from low-resource, agrarian socialist countries to relatively high-resource, industrialized capitalist societies.

16.8.2 Emergency Management Mission Area

The CDC program's goals mandated the mission area for emergency response. This CDC program assisted partnering national health ministries to write provincial-level EOPs that would be implemented by health ministries with the support of multiple other public and private sectors. These EOPs would be executed immediately in response to the ongoing public health emergency in southeast Asia.

16.8.3 Functional Analysis

A functional analysis of pandemic emergency response was performed based upon the following sources: (a) robust models of currently-existing national-level pandemic response plans (e.g., USA and Australia) and (b) a review of the world English scientific literature regarding pandemic preparedness (e.g., WHO and CDC guidance for pandemic preparedness and response, journal articles, and organizational websites). The results of this review were then stored in one common database called "the library." Different versions of the library (referred to as "books") were selected through a partner country review. Finally, each country then revised these "books" to become "plans." Each plan was then presented in a software format that was most useful to that nation.

Figure 16.3 illustrates the process used for the functional analysis of pandemic response operations.

16.8.4 Capability Inventory

Table 16.1 lists the eighteen core capabilities for pandemic emergency operations identified through functional analysis of existing information.

These eighteen pandemic response capabilities were compiled (in association with their respective goals, objectives, and activities) into a relational database called "the library." This database was represented on the following two separate platforms: (1) a **Microsoft Excel™ spreadsheet** (.xls) operating from a local hard drive and (2) a **Microsoft SQL Server™ database** (.xml) operating from a remote server (i.e., "in the cloud").

Given this listing of eighteen core response capabilities, plan stakeholders in each country were convened to review individual, country-specific templates (i.e., "books") containing these capabilities to identify which of these capabilities were applicable in each

Table 16.1 Eighteen core capabilities of pandemic influenza emergency response operations identified by functional analysis of existing publications

1. animal related issues
2. antiviral distribution and use
3. clinical management
4. command and control
5. community disease control and prevention
6. ethical issues
7. fatality management
8. healthcare operations
9. isolation and quarantine
10. laboratory services
11. medical supply management
12. operational communications
13. policy issues
14. psychosocial support
15. risk communication
16. surveillance
17. travel related risk of disease transmission
18. vaccine distribution and use

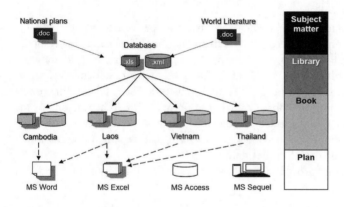

Figure 16.3 Functional analysis of pandemic emergency operations from existing publications

jurisdiction. The result was that all four nations felt that they had the ability to accomplish all eighteen response capabilities. Simply stated, each nation also chose to aggregate these eighteen core capabilities into a handful of larger functional elements. For example, given their unique set of needs and resources, Thailand summarized these eighteen core capabilities into the following six functional elements: command and control; livestock preparedness; public health preparedness; communication and public relations; transportation and cross border issues; and security and relief. In comparison, Laos chose to aggregate these same eighteen capabilities into the following five functional elements: coordination and decision-making; surveillance and reporting; public health measures; essential health services; and communication.

Each country also made individualized decisions regarding the final platform for the plan itself. As illustrated at the bottom in Figure 16.3, Cambodia preferred the plan's final format to be an easily reviewable and widely accessible word document (e.g., **MS Word**™ **word processor**). Laos also preferred this same narrative document format in addition to a version in spreadsheet format. In comparison, both Vietnam and Thailand developed and presented their final plan in spreadsheet-format-only (Microsoft Excel™ spreadsheet) to quickly be revised and shared via email. None of the four nations utilized database software (e.g., **Microsoft Access**™ **database**) or data networking across multiple **servers** (e.g., Microsoft SQL Server™) (see Figure 16.3).

16.9 Questions for Discussion

Briefly describe how you would utilize Tables 4.1–4.3 to perform a functional analysis and capability inventory for a public health agency response to flooding.

a. What are the health hazards?
b. What are the health consequences?
c. What are the needs caused by the consequences?
d. What are the capabilities needed to address those needs?

Chapter

17

Risk Assessment

17.1 Learning Objectives

Upon completion of the chapter, the reader can:

1. Define the following terms and phrases:
   - ADEPT™ risk assessment decision tree
   - Disability
   - Disaster-related health risk
   - Disaster risk
   - Dose rate
   - Dose–response modeling
   - Hazard analysis
   - Hazard characterization
   - Hazard identification
   - Hazard map
   - Hazard prioritization
   - Health hazard
   - Health risk
   - Impact analysis
   - Index
   - Morbidity
   - Mortality
   - Pathophysiologic
   - Prevalence
   - Prevalent
   - Risk
   - Risk characterization
   - Risk equation
   - Risk management
   - Scale
   - Susceptibility
   - Uncertainty
   - Vulnerability.

2. List the three steps involved in the assessment of planning assumptions.
3. List the three main components of a risk assessment.
4. Compare and contrast the risk of disaster incidence, $p(D)$, with that of disaster-related health risk, $p(DH)$.

5. List the two stages of hazard analysis.
6. Identify a low probability–high impact event using a hazard probability matrix figure.
7. Describe the two key clusters of disaster-related health consequences.
8. Write the "risk equation" used for calculating disaster-related health risk, $p(D_H)$.
9. Compare and contrast reliability and validity.
10. Compare and contrast the use of scales and indices for data measurement.
11. Use the ADEPT™ risk assessment decision tree to perform a rapid risk assessment:

- With historical data available, with risk expressed as a scale.
- Without data available, with risk expressed as an index.

17.2 Risk

In its simplest terms, **risk** is the probability that a specific outcome will occur (out of all possible outcomes). This outcome may be beneficial or adverse. This relationship may be represented as: $p(\text{risk}) = \int p(\text{outcome})$ [34, 69].

Risk represents the effect of uncertainty on outcomes
– ISO 31000

Uncertainty is a state or condition that involves a deficiency of information and leads to inadequate or incomplete knowledge or understanding [40]. Uncertainty exists whenever the knowledge or understanding of an event, consequence, or likelihood is inadequate or incomplete [40]. Statistical uncertainty is often calculated as the interval around the measurement in which repeated measurements will fall. Therefore, expressions of risk should include estimations of uncertainty as follows: $p(\text{risk}) = \int p(\text{outcome}) \pm \text{uncertainty}$ [34].

Risk represents future events that have not yet occurred. Once an event occurs, it is no longer considered a risk. Instead, it is referred to as an "incident." In public health, this occurrence is referred to as "incidence." It is commonly represented as the rate or proportion of an adverse health outcome. In epidemiology, "incidence" refers to the occurrence of new disease cases (including injury) in a population over a specified period.

In comparison to disease incidence, a disease is prevalent when it is present among a particular population (over a specific area, or during a specified period). **Prevalence** (sometimes referred to as prevalence rate) is "the proportion of persons in a population who have a particular disease or attribute at a specified point in time or over a specified period" [70].

Prevention is used to reduce disease occurrence – (incidence)
Treatment is added to reduce disease progression – (prevalence)

This relationship is described as follows in what is commonly referred to as the **risk equation**: $p(\text{R}) = \int p(\text{H} \times \text{I}) \pm \text{uncertainty}$, where R = risk; H = hazard incidence; and I = degree of impact [71].

As introduced in Chapter 2, hazards are defined as "... an agent or a situation ... with the inherent capability to have an adverse effect" [72]. Risk is the joint probability that (in the future): (1) one of these hazards will occur and (2) there will be a resultant impact. Thus, to accurately predict risk, it is first necessary to describe the outcome in terms that are specific and measurable (i.e., consistent with Doran's SMART objectives discussed in Section 8.9). In other words, we must first ask, "What risk are we assessing?" This question sounds simple enough, but misconceptions related to disaster risk are all too common.

While there are now multiple examples of qualitative and semi-quantitative "risk assessments" being used for some degree of predicting disaster-related health risk, few models express health risk in terms of the actual probability of outcomes, along with uncertainty (the very definition of risk, according to the ISO 31000) [73]. This then complicates the ability to prioritize and allocate capacity effectively.

17.3 Disaster Risk

In the case of disasters and health, part of this confusion appears to stem from the lack of differentiation between the probability of disasters and the probability of disaster-related *health effects*. More specifically, **disaster risk**, $p(D)$, is defined as the "probability of harmful consequences, or expected losses (deaths, injuries, property, livelihoods, economic activity disrupted or environment damaged) resulting from interactions between natural or human-induced hazards and vulnerable conditions" [74, p. 9]. It is considered as "the potential loss of life, injury, or destroyed or damaged assets which could occur to a system, society or a community in a specific period, determined probabilistically as a function of hazard, exposure, vulnerability and capacity" [75, p. 9].

Disaster risk, $p(D)$, is thus defined as the probability of a characteristic mismatch of societal needs and resources as an outcome. In comparison, health risk is defined as the probability of adverse health outcomes. Disaster risk, therefore, differs from disaster-related health risk in that (by definition) disaster risk is a measure of not only the probability of adverse outcomes (i.e., all impacts, including health) but also the capacity, $p(C)$, of the society at large to avoid a mismatch of needs (caused by losses) and resources. To summarize [34]:

- Hazards create damage or losses (e.g., disease).
  - o The severity of losses is expressed in terms of impact.

- Impacts create needs.
  - o Abilities required to meet these needs are expressed in terms of capabilities.

- Capabilities meet needs.
  - o The measure of a capability that is available over time is expressed in terms of capacity.

17.4 Disaster-Related Health Risk

Disaster-related health risk occurs as a result of direct or indirect exposure to **health hazards**. Health hazards are defined as an agent or a situation that, when exposed to a human, has the inherent capability to cause an adverse health outcome (disease), resulting in **morbidity** (illness or injury), **mortality** (death), and/or **disability** [72]. For this reason, it is important to carefully scrutinize the applicability of so-called health-related "hazard-vulnerability analyses" or "vulnerability indices" constructed to model the risk of a *disaster* compared to the risk of disaster-related *health effects* as the specific and measurable outcome.

The epidemiological definition of **health risk**, $p(R_H)$, is the "probability that an adverse health event will occur" (e.g., that an individual will become ill or die within a stated period or age) [76]. It is formally defined as the "proportion of initially disease-free individuals who develop a disease over a defined period of observation" [70]. This risk is described in terms of disease incidence rate or proportion (e.g., the measure of the number of new cases per unit of time) [34].

When applied to public health, health risk is the probability that, in a certain timeframe, an adverse outcome will occur among a population that is exposed to a hazardous agent. Disease is caused by the complex interaction of risk and protective factors associated with health determinants [34].

When applied to disasters, **disaster-related health risk**, $p(D_H)$, can be described as the probability of disease, given a disaster has occurred. Thus, $p(D_H) = p(R_H) \mid p(D) = 1$. Thus, disaster-related health risk, $p(D_H)$, is often expressed as the annual disaster-related case incidence rate and described as the proportion of individuals within a given population (and over a defined time) who experience morbidity and mortality: (1) due to direct hazard exposure and (2) due to a mismatch of community needs and resources caused by the disaster hazard.

Figure 17.1 depicts the relationship between the direct and indirect causes of disaster-related health effects.

According to the transitive property, disaster-related health risk is therefore expressed in terms of:

- p(Disaster-related health risk) $= p$(Disaster hazard) $\times p$(health impact); or
- p(Disaster-related health risk) $= p$(Disaster hazard) $\times p$(health needs $-$ health resources); or
- p(Disaster-related health risk) $= p$(hazard) $\times [p$(vulnerability $\times$ exposure) $- p$(capacity)].

Thus, the risk equation is applied to estimate disaster-related health risk as follows:

$$p(D_H) = \int [p(H) \times p[E \times V] - p(C)]. \quad [77]$$

17.5 Risk Assessment

Risk assessment is the process of estimating the probability of an outcome under a specific set of conditions and for a certain timeframe (in this case, the impact of a hazardous agent

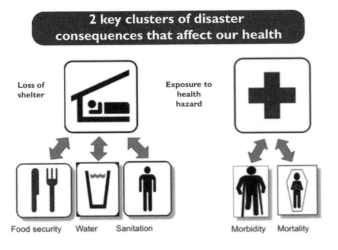

Figure 17.1 The two key clusters of disaster-related health consequences

on a specified human population). Thus, health risk assessments express risk in terms of the probability of a specific health outcome. They also include an estimation of the degree of uncertainty related to this assessment.

This book aims to create effective emergency operations plans (EOPs) for the public health and medical sector. Accordingly, our risk assessments focus on the public health and medical consequences for which this sector holds significant response capability, in other words, on disaster-related health risk.

Risk assessments typically consist of the following three main components: (1) **hazard analysis,** (2) **impact analysis,** and (3) **risk characterization.**

Hazard analyses typically include two stages: hazard identification and hazard characterization. Hazard identification involves recognition of those hazards that are likely to occur within a given location. Hazard characterization involves identifying the frequency of those hazards, and then describing the adverse health effects that may result from exposure to the hazard [78, 79].

Impact analysis seeks to quantify the degree of damage or losses (e.g., disease) that may be expected when a vulnerable population is exposed to a hazard. For health, these potential losses include disaster-related morbidity and mortality. Impact analysis, therefore, includes an assessment of those risk factors besides hazard, which are known to influence disaster-related health outcomes (i.e., exposures, vulnerability, and capacity) [77].

Risks characterizations are used to combine the various factors affecting disaster-related disease (i.e., hazards, exposure, vulnerability, and capacity) into one measure of joint probability. This characterization allows for a standardized comparison among a wide variety of disaster risks. Risk characterizations described in this book focus on the probability of disaster-related morbidity and mortality as indicators of disaster-related health risk.

17.6 Hazard Analysis

17.6.1 Hazard Identification

Hazard analyses typically include two stages: **hazard identification** and **hazard characterization.** Hazard analyses begin by identifying all hazards that can affect a given jurisdiction (e.g., institution, city, state, or nation). During hazard characterization, the relative probability (i.e., likelihood of future occurrence) is then estimated for each of the hazards, using historical records and scientific hazard prediction modeling whenever available. **Hazard maps** are also routinely created to depict the relative probability of critical hazards according to geographical location.

In the US, this information is readily available as the National Risk Index, a new, online mapping application from the Federal Emergency Management Agency (i.e., FEMA) that identifies communities most at risk to eighteen natural hazards. This application visualizes natural hazard risk metrics and includes data about expected annual losses, social vulnerabilities, and community resilience [80].

The information regarding "expected annual loss" is derived from multiple institutions' data and is remarkably accurate. This risk factor also includes calculations for both hazard likelihood, $p(H)$, and exposure, $p(E)$. However, it should be noted that assumptions regarding the quantifiable relationships between vulnerability and resilience, as noted in the National Risk Index data, remain mostly theoretical and unvalidated. Therefore, these approaches are not yet recommended as a first choice for predicting disaster-related health risk, $p(D_H)$, as compared to the likelihood of disaster, $p(D)$.

Finally, we should consider that the three factors of the National Risk Index (i.e., expected annual loss, social vulnerability, and community resilience) are intended to predict the risk of disaster, $p(D)$, and not the risk of adverse health effects, given that a disaster has occurred, i.e., $\left(p(D_H) \mid p(D) = 1 \right)$. For this reason, this book recommends using the US National Risk Index for hazard and exposure data only.

For nations other than the United States, the Prevention Web disaster and risk profiles are an excellent source of readily available, standardized risk information for individual nations that may also be compared as a reference [81]. This information includes both hazard and impact data that can often be used as another alternative method for risk assessment. It is advantageous in the case of low resource countries where standardized data may be otherwise unavailable. In this case, this book recommends utilizing the Prevention Web risk indices in place of (or in addition to) subjective risk estimates made in the absence of historical data.

17.6.2 Hazard Characterization

Capability-based planning involves a functional analysis of critical operational requirements [55, 82]. Once hazards are identified, this functional analysis is performed to describe the specific impact being considered. For the health sector, this impact is commonly represented in terms of morbidity and mortality [78, 79]. Functional analysis typically divides a system into smaller parts, called functional elements, which describe "*what*" we want each part to do. It does not include the "*how*" or solution yet. This parsing allows for the same functional analysis to be used by differing stakeholders for the same hazards. Tables 4.1–4.3 offer a standardized approach for the functional analysis and characterization of disaster-related health hazards in the case of public health emergencies. This process is known as descriptive characterization and serves to structure information associated with a particular hazard and how the host and the environment influence it. Thus a hazard characterization for one particular hazard may offer a standard building block for risk assessments conducted for various purposes [82].

Disaster hazard characterization begins with assessing the public health consequences and relative impacts (see Tables 4.1 and 4.2) and then progresses to identify the corresponding core capabilities (i.e., functional elements) needed for each disaster hazard identified (see Table 4.3).

In this sense, the process of hazard characterization is a functional analysis applied to the impacts of disaster-related health hazards.

Tables 4.1–4.3 offer a standard template for hazard characterization using functional analysis of the public health and medical sectors (including natural and technological hazards). Tables 4.1 and 4.2 provide an overview of the public health consequences addressed by thirty-two categories of public health and medical functions [21]. Table 4.3 then lists the public health capabilities necessary to address those public health consequences listed in Tables 4.1 and 4.2 that are most commonly addressed in disaster response [21]. Plan stakeholders may refer to this functional analysis for the public health and medical sector as they: (1) anticipate the public health consequences and needs associated with all disaster hazards and (2) document their own institutional ability to address the needs (i.e., capability inventory).

The hierarchical tree of the ADEPT™ system serves as a practical framework for guiding functional analysis. It divides the plan into cascading functional elements (e.g., capabilities, goals, objectives, and activities) and their related material and human resources.

Within public health, capabilities are typically divided according to sub-disciplines (e.g., infectious disease, environmental health, injury prevention and control, occupational health and safety, chronic disease, maternal–child health, global health, laboratory, epidemiology). Within healthcare, capabilities are commonly divided according to outpatient clinical specialty (e.g., internal medicine, pediatrics, surgery, mental health, nursing) or inpatient hospital department (e.g., triage, emergency, radiology, laboratory, wards, surgery, isolation, intensive care, morgue).

17.7 Impact Analysis

Impact is a measure of outcome [74]. The incidence of disease is one example of a measure of disaster-related health outcome and thus one measure of disaster impact. Health impact (I_H) is expressed as a rate and measured in terms of disease incidence resulting from exposure and vulnerability to a particular hazard, minus any losses that may be ameliorated by applying capacity. In other words, when a disaster hazard occurs, $p(H)$, it creates an impact, $p(I)$, that also affects the likelihood of disaster-related health risk, $p(D_H)$. Thus, $p(I_H) = \int[p(E \times V) - p(C)]$, where $p(I_H)$ = health impact; E = exposure dose; V = vulnerability of population, and C = capacity to respond (in a manner that reduces adverse health outcomes). In simple terms, risk occurs as a result of both hazards and impact. The impacts of health hazards are customarily assessed according to factors associated with the interaction between the agent, environment, and the host population (respectively), as follows [82]:

- Hazardous agent – the range and character of **pathophysiologic** effects, given hazard exposure;
- Exposure dose – the amount of hazard contacted over time (**dose rate**), given hazard incidence; and
- Population vulnerability – the relative **susceptibility** to disease incidence or progression given hazard exposure.

Exposures are assessed for each of the hazards identified in the initial hazard analysis. Exposures are assessed in terms of dose. This dose rate represents the relative magnitude of the hazard and its contact rate for the population over time. When exposure data are available, the hazard analysis also includes quantitative information regarding the dose–response relationship (the relationship between hazard dose and health response) and the probability of adverse outcomes through dose reconstruction and **dose–response modeling** [77, 82, 83].

When data is available, exposure is best expressed as a range of potential minimum and maximum dose values that better describe variation and the potential for extremes than representations of central tendency. Dose–response modeling represents the relationship between exposure to the hazard and subsequent health effects among the population. In the future, the same could potentially be accomplished for all-natural and technological disaster hazards.

17.8 Risk Characterization

Once the hazard and impact analyses are complete, this information is used to guide overall disaster risk characterization. Risk characterization calculates the joint probability of hazard probability and their impacts, $p(H) \times p(I)$, and then prioritizes these disaster hazards according to overall disaster-related health risk, $p(D_H)$. This risk is described in terms of the joint probability of the hazard and its subsequent impact. The risk is then ranked according to this priority.

When numerical data are available, disaster-related health risk, $p(D_H)$, and ratio scales may be calculated and compared among differing hazards. When such data is unavailable, the risk is characterized as an index and is commonly represented as a hazard probability impact matrix.

Figure 17.2 provides an example of a simple hazard probability-impact matrix. High probability / high impact events (noted in the right upper corner of Figure 17.2) are given the most priority, while low probability / low impact events (depicted in the bottom left corner of Figure 17.2) are given the least priority. This prioritization is often depicted in a **hazard-impact matrix**, with probability represented on the *y*-axis and impact represented on the *x*-axis.

17.9 Risk Management

Ideally, emergency management is based on a ***risk prioritization*** process. Risk assessments are used to provide disaster planners with actionable intelligence for this use in this prioritization. Once hazards have been identified, they are assessed in terms of their probability. And their impact is assessed in terms of losses. The hazards associated with the most significant probability and impact are prioritized. In addition to prioritization, risk assessment also offers a process for ongoing research involving the interaction of health determinants, risk, and protective factors that may alter future adverse health outcomes. Finally, risk assessment provides a framework for monitoring and evaluating the performance of **risk management** interventions intended to reduce adverse health outcomes [77].

17.10 Risk Assessment for Disaster-Related Health Outcomes

The utility of existing health-related disaster risk assessment models is often attenuated by challenges with both first- and second-order uncertainty. This uncertainty is often due to a

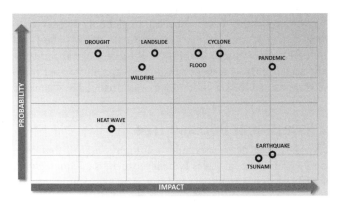

Figure 17.2 Probability-impact matrix for natural disaster hazards

lack of predictability (reflected in the standard deviation) and accuracy (reflected in the standard error) of these assessments. This absence of metrics has limited the utility of most public health disaster risk assessments. This uncertainty logically results in acceptably accurate hazard identification and prioritization but inaccurate and nonreproducible estimations of health-related impact [77].

As a result, three main approaches are proposed for improving assessment utility. The first two approaches differ in that they use different ordinal measures to represent the information as either a **scale** or an **index**. The third approach uses capability-based planning (as discussed in Section 9.4), a different approach to overcome uncertainty.

Typically, both scales and indices employ multiple observations or items of measurement. However, in risk assessment for disaster-related disease, indices that lack quantitative values are not based upon empirical measures but somewhat subjective estimates that are more prone to first- and second-order uncertainty. For example, the root causes of disaster-related health risk (i.e., exposure, vulnerability, and capacity) are typically estimated using a relatively imprecise ordinal index or ranking (e.g., "very high, high, moderate, low, very low"). This index is usually a composite of unproven assumptions regarding the causal pathways of disaster-related health risk.

Some risk assessment models offer indices derived from semi-quantitative estimates of select disaster risk components (namely hazards, vulnerability, and capacity). Other models offer a retrospective analysis of the association between disaster incidence and select risk factors (e.g., social vulnerability and capacity) [77, 84–86].

Thus, most tools used to assess disaster-related disease lack predictive value that would guide accurate cost accounting necessary to justify large-scale resource allocation or investment.

In comparison to the use of risk indices, ratio scales have also been used to describe the risk of disaster-related disease. These scales focus on describing one measurable outcome (e.g., the probability of disaster-related health impact, $p(I_H)$). This impact is then expressed using specific and measurable public health indicators (e.g., morbidity and mortality rates). And while the uncertainty of these values may remain relatively high due to a lack of predictability (reflected in the standard deviation), accuracy (reflected in the standard error) is improved using this scale, as compared to an ordinal index of subjective estimates. This accuracy results in improved reliability of the assessment. A numerical scale also allows for statistical calculations and statements that describe the relative degree of uncertainty. This calculation is not possible using ordinal indices.

Finally (as discussed in Section 9.4), if disaster data is not available to adequately inform either an ordinal estimate of risk index or a numerical calculation of risk using a scale, disaster planners may then also apply a capability-based approach to planning that serves to compensate for the relatively high degree of uncertainty. This unpredictability is best met by planning to accomplish those objectives within our ability to achieve (i.e., capability) – rather than the constraints of the scenario. In emergency response, capability-based planning allows for the flexibility necessary to address a wide range of unpredictable scenarios.

17.11 The ADEPT™ Risk Assessment Decision Tree

This book offers a framework for assessing disaster-related health risk, $p(D_H)$, that integrates the use of risk indices along with numerical scales (whenever there is adequate data).

Figure 17.3 depicts the ADEPT™ risk assessment decision tree is an algorithm that may be used for assessing disaster-related health risk. This algorithm includes two main

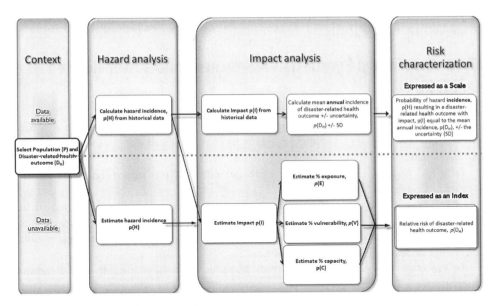

Figure 17.3 The ADEPT™ risk assessment decision tree

pathways. The top one is expressed as a scale and the bottom one as an index. The pathway is decided based upon the availability of health data related to each specific disaster hazard. In the upper pathway, data is available. In the lower pathway, data is not. In all cases, calculations of central tendency and variance (i.e., means and standard deviation) are preferable to subjective estimates of relative degrees of impact.

Risk assessment begins by deciding the context for the assessment. This context includes selecting the specific target population (P) to be served and the specific disaster-related health outcome being studied (D_H). Then, depending upon historical hazard data availability, the assessor either calculates or estimates the hazard's annual incidence, $p(H)$. This probability is usually expressed as an annual percentage or as a "100-year event."

Then, depending upon the availability of historical impact data (e.g., hazard-specific disease incidence), the assessor either calculates or estimates the mean annual disease incidence, $p(D_H)$. When data is available, this risk of disaster-related disease, $p(D_H)$, is expressed as a ratio scale. This scale then characterizes the risk of disaster-related disease as the annual percent-probability of a hazard that would result in a health impact of average size for that hazard.

Where data is unavailable, the causal factors of disaster-related health outcomes (i.e., exposure, **vulnerability**, and capacity) are instead estimated and combined to be expressed as a relative index. This index broadly characterizes disaster-related disease risk along a semi-quantitative scale (e.g., very low, low, moderate, high, and very high). This scale is used to describe the risk applied to both the hazard incidence and its associated impact (e.g., "low probability – high impact"). The risk may then be compared for different hazards using a probability-impact matrix (see Figure 17.2).

Finally, the risk is characterized as the joint probability of the hazard and its impact. When data is available, this is the probability of hazard incidence, $p(H)$, resulting in a disaster-related health outcome with impact, $p(I)$, equal to the mean annual incidence of disaster-related disease, $p(D_H)$.

17.12 Case Study: Pyronesia's Assessment of Disaster-Related Health Risk

Let us now consider a case study using the ADEPT™ risk assessment algorithm. The nation of Pyronesia has mandated the updating of its public health EOP. As part of an assessment of planning assumptions, Pyronesian planners have decided to perform a national risk assessment.

Table 17.1 reveals the results of a risk characterization performed for significant disaster hazards in Pyronesia

Like the rest of the world, floods are among the most common disasters in Pyronesia, and data are, therefore, more readily available than other disaster hazards. So, planners have chosen to assess the risk for flood-related morbidity and mortality among a target population that includes all the people of Pyronesia.

As expected, Pyronesia can draw from historical records to find the mean annual likelihood for a flood hazard occurrence that resulted in a disaster declaration, $p(H)$. In any given year, there is a 10 percent likelihood of a flood-related disaster declaration.

Also, in Pyronesia, there are good records that describe the morbidity and mortality related to flood events over the past 100 years. So, the mean annual rates of disaster-related morbidity and mortality are also available. Rapid epidemiological needs assessments performed after flood disasters reveal mean annual morbidity of 74 ± 88 and mean annual mortality of 140 ± 227. Thus, the disaster-related health risk, $p(D_H)$, due to flood may be

Table 17.1. Disaster hazards characterized in order of descending risk for Pyronesia

Priority	Hazard
1	Human epidemic
2	Severe storms Road crash
3	Rail crash
4	Animal epidemic Industrial fire Infrastructure failure
5	Dangerous goods spill Explosions Terrorism Stampede
6	Flood Urban fire
7	Dam failure
8	Wildland fire Landslide

presented as a ratio scale as follows: In any given year, there is a 10 percent risk of flooding that will result in 74 ± 88 (e.g., range = 0–162) illnesses and 140 ± 227 (e.g., range = 0–367) deaths. Pyronesia may then use this data as actionable intelligence when considered within the context of national capabilities available to manage <100 illnesses and <400 deaths per year. Subsequent functional analyses and capability inventories reveal that Pyronesia has the internal capacity to respond to most flood disasters and will most likely not require external assistance. They may also plan specific response measures on a scale commensurate with the risk (as opposed to the worst-case scenario). Worst-case scenarios and deliberately conservative estimates reduce the risk assessment's utility for cost-benefit studies and uncertainty descriptions [82].

Now, let us consider an example of a different hazard with less data availability (e.g., earthquake). Despite historical accounts of a major earthquake that occurred a millennia ago, Pyronesia has no modern record of an earthquake disaster. While useful seismic and geological data are available for predicting the likelihood of future earthquakes (e.g., annual $p(H) = 0.1$ percent), there is no historical information available to predict the health impacts of such an event in modern times. In this case, Pyronesia may choose to utilize these quantitative hazard predictions along with a more subjective estimate of health impact based upon extrapolations of factors observed in similar events that have occurred elsewhere (e.g., exposure, vulnerability, and capacity) to predict the overall disaster-related health risk, $p(D_H)$.

For example, they may choose to estimate the risk of exposure as the 40 percent of the national population that lives in the seismically active region located in the country's northeast edge.

The target population may also estimate the population's vulnerability based upon demographic and public health data that includes age, gender, socio-economic status, household composition, and health status. This likelihood of vulnerability is estimated to comprise 50 percent of the target population (or 20 percent of the nation).

Given the proportion of the nation's population living in the region and then the size of that sub-component of that most vulnerable population, estimates of health outcomes (e.g., morbidity and mortality) are then made. Considering the relatively lethal nature of earthquake hazards (up to 50 percent case fatality rates have been reported) and that 20 percent of the nation is both exposed and vulnerable, these impacts are predicted to result in high morbidity and mortality rates in Pyronesia.

Thus, the disaster-related health risk, $p(D_H)$, due to an earthquake may be estimated as an ordinal index as follows: In any given year, there is a 0.1 percent risk of an earthquake that will result in a high number of injuries and a high number of deaths. This is described as a "low probability–high impact event" with a moderately-high degree of uncertainty.

Once the potential health impact is identified, Pyronesia may perform a functional analysis to identify what functions (and their associated capabilities) will be needed to respond in a way that will reduce that morbidity and mortality. As indicated in Table 4.1, there are typically many severely injured victims in the case of earthquakes. Thus, the functional analysis would expectedly identify the need for prehospital and hospital-based trauma care. Subsequent capability assessments would also expectedly identify trauma care capabilities and inventory their capacity. Any gaps are then mandated as the focus of operational objectives included in the national preparedness plan.

Finally, there is the possibility that some jurisdictions may be at significant risk for low probability–high impact events for which there are no data available for either the hazard or

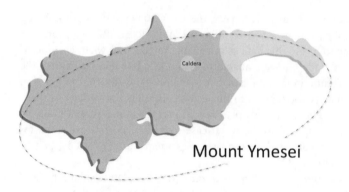

Figure 17.4 The remnants of ancient volcano, Mount Ymesei

its impact. For example, scientists have only recently discovered that Caldera, the capitol of Pyronesia, is located over Mount Ymesei, a dormant (but not extinct) volcano magma chamber not previously recognized (see Figure 17.4).

At this time, there are little historical or scientific data available regarding the likelihood of this disaster hazard or its potential health impact. Therefore, the Pyronesian public health disaster planners must estimate both hazard and impact values to obtain an index of relative risk that may compare to other disaster hazards for prioritization. Thus, the disaster-related health risk, $p(D_H)$, due to volcanic eruption may be described as follows: In any given year, there is a very low risk of a volcanic eruption that will result in a very high number of injuries and a very high number of deaths (mostly in the densely populated capitol city). This risk is described as a "very low probability–very high impact event" with a high degree of uncertainty.

17.13 Questions for Discussion

1. Rank the following disaster hazards according to probability and impact in Pyronesia as either high, medium, or low. Justify your answers.

Hazard	Probability	Impact	Rank
Terrorist attack			
Tsunami			
Ice storm			
Train crash			

2. Describe how risk assessment involving terrorism threats differ from that for natural and human-made hazards in that they involve an estimation of intent and technical capability.
3. Describe why developing a national preparedness program for very low probability–very high impact events can be particularly challenging.

Creating Plans

18.1 Learning Objectives

Upon completion of the chapter, the reader can:

1. Define the following terms and phrases:
   • Preparedness plan for response (PPR).
2. List the four steps for creating an EOP.
3. List the six steps of plan-writing.
4. List the four steps for creating a preparedness plan.
5. Describe the process for integrating an EOP with its associated preparedness plan.

18.2 Emergency Operations Planning

Figure 18.1 depicts the second phase in the ADEPT™ planning system, creating a mission area plan (an emergency operations plan (EOP) for the response mission area). At first, it may appear counterintuitive that we are writing a plan for emergency response before writing a preparedness plan. However, by identifying and stating the activities necessary if an emergency were to occur today, it then becomes possible to identify any gaps in

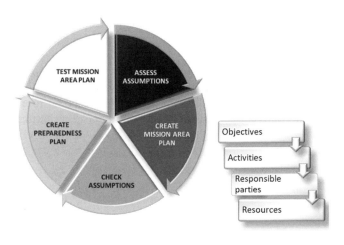

Figure 18.1 Four steps for creating an EOP, as the second phase of the planning wheel

capability or capacity that may be predicted for the future. We then use the preparedness plan to design a system that addresses the gaps between our current capacity and the capacity predicted to be needed in the event of a disaster.

During this process, stakeholders use consensus-based group decision-making and follow the SOARR™ format to draft strategic goals, operational objectives, and activities that accomplish those objectives. Finally, they assign responsible parties and other resources for each related activity. These resources have typically included estimates of time, personnel, financing, and essential elements of information in the past.

As introduced in Table 1.1, strategic goals serve as a standard model of quality related to capability. Operational objectives serve as a standard model of quality related to the effectiveness of outcomes. And finally, activities and resources serve as a standard model of quality related to performance efficiency.

18.3 Creating an EOP

18.3.1 The O2C3 Model

As introduced in Section 6.2, the ADEPT™ planning system uses an "O2C3" model to combine five approaches for effective planning (e.g., operational-level, objective-based, capability-based, consensus-based, and compliant with population norms and regulations) [13, 21, 25, 27, 28, 50].

In other words, using this system, stakeholders may apply the principles of consensus-based group decision-making to create an objective-based EOP that (1) describes their capability in terms of emergency operations and (2) is compliant with applicable norms.

This approach is best implemented through the use of a group facilitator. The facilitator's role is to support and empower the stakeholders' work as a neutral broker in the planning process. Facilitators help to recognize rules of order and manage the group's expectations for a productive outcome. It is also helpful to use a transcriptionist to assist the facilitator, whose role is to enter and manipulate the spreadsheet data for group viewing.

18.3.2 The SOARR™ Format

The creation of an EOP begins with the results of a capability inventory. A list of capabilities is derived from this inventory. A SOARR™ table is then created for each capability listed in the inventory (see Table 18.1).

State and national-level EOPs typically contain between ten and thirty strategic goals. Each strategic goal is then ideally comprised of three-to-five operational objectives that accomplish the strategic goal. For each operational objective, there should be no more than ten activities. (If there are more offered, plan facilitators should consider splitting

Table 18.1. SOARR™ format table for emergency planning

Strategic goal	Operational objective	Activity	Responsible party	Resource

the operational objective into sub-components.) There should be only one party assigned to be primarily responsible for ensuring and reporting its completion to the incident command system for each activity. There can be multiple supporting roles that are listed as secondarily responsible. Resources should also be identified and assigned to every activity.

In many cases, the strategic goals, operational objectives, and even most activities can be drafted by an experienced public health planner or incident manager in advance of all EOP stakeholders' convening together. This preparation can save time since stakeholders do not have to create the language of the plan de novo. They may instead review and edit the language as a group. The following six steps then accomplish plan-writing during the group meeting:

1. The facilitator reads the proposed entry aloud, and
2. the facilitator asks if this entry is applicable. If not, it is deleted.
3. If applicable, the facilitator asks if it is stated correctly.
4. The facilitator then moderates the subsequent group discussion of the entry.
5. The facilitator moderates the group editing of the entry wording.
6. The facilitator reads the final entry together with the group.

These six steps are repeated for each empty box in the SOARR™ format table (see Figure 18.1). Entries are ALWAYS reviewed and edited in order – line by line starting from left to right (i.e., beginning with the strategic goal and continuing to the right until all corresponding objectives, activities, responsible parties, and resources have been completed). The same process is then repeated for each capability until the entire EOP is completed.

Previous studies of the process have revealed that (once initiated) stakeholders can plan at a rate averaging at fifteen objectives per hour and up to thirty activities per hour. This rate is also associated with a high degree of participant satisfaction during the process [27]. This has allowed entire communities to write a sixty-page-long EOP in less than fifteen hours.

Over the years, stakeholder revisions have also been studied extensively. It may be said that when presented with a pre-written EOP, the level of stakeholder revision tends to increase moving across the SOARR™ format table from left to right. Stakeholders do not tend to make significant changes in the strategic goals, and their edits are usually limited to about 20 percent of pre-drafted operational objectives. Stakeholders also typically edit around 50 percent of pre-drafted activities, and, of course, all responsible parties are unique to each EOP, so stakeholders typically assign 100 percent of responsibilities and resources in the absence of pre-drafted suggestions.

18.4 Creating a Preparedness Plan for Response (PPR)

Figure 18.2 depicts the fourth step in the ADEPT™ planning wheel, creating the preparedness plan.

Preparedness planning for response (PPR) is intended to build capacity and capabilities necessary for effective management of any mission area, including emergency response. Measures of success for the mission area of emergency response are derived from the EOP itself. Once gaps in capability or capacity have been identified, the preparedness

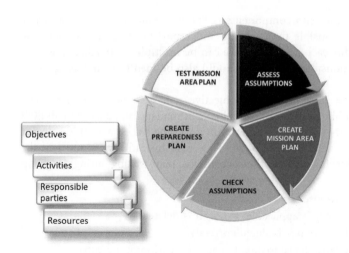

Figure 18.2 Steps for creating a preparedness plan, as the fourth phase of the planning wheel

plan details the objectives, activities, responsible parties, and timeline for resolving this operational deficiency.

In this sense, mission area plans (e.g., EOPs) and PPRs must be directly connected. PPRs focus on filling the gaps that have been found to exist in mission area plans. Public health preparedness programs may apply this focus toward measurable gains in capability or capacity to influence health outcomes. Thus, the EOP serves as the standard model for acceptable performance, and the PPR serves as the means to meet that standard and improve future performance.

Creating a mission area plan without a preparedness plan is like taking the final exam without taking the class

Figure 18.3 illustrates how the SOARR™ format used for mission area plans integrates into the preparedness cycle, as introduced in Figure 2.1.

As mentioned in Chapter 2, it is notable that the preparedness cycle is based upon a hybrid version of the Deming cycle (Plan–Do–Check–Act) for quality control and Fayol's five functions of management. In other words, the preparedness cycle applies Deming's quality control loop and Fayol's five functions of management to each activity of the mission area plan.

These preparedness plans begin with the same strategic goals and operational objectives as the associated EOP. In many cases, those identified as responsible for individual activities in the EOP are also the most appropriate persons to accomplish the preparedness plan's capacity-building activities. However, the activities and resources needed for preparedness are usually different than those needed for response. Therefore, it is necessary to write a preparedness plan that addresses each of the gaps in capacity identified during the intervening gap analysis. Thus, the preparedness plan describes a system for quality control applied to managing tactical

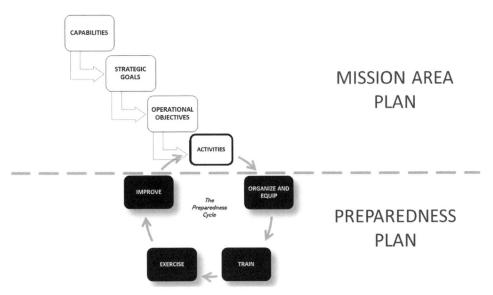

Figure 18.3 Integration of mission area plans with preparedness plans

operations described in the EOP (e.g., specific activities and their associated resourcing). Once an EOP is created, the preparedness plan then describes operations (i.e., a set of processes) that organize/equip, train, exercise, and improve each activity in the EOP. Put simply, these five elements of the preparedness cycle could also be represented as the predicate "O-T-E-I" following SOARR™ stated in the EOP (see Figure 18.1). In other words, the entire preparedness plan is comprised of SOARR™ data from the EOP aligned with corresponding "OTEI" data from the preparedness cycle.

As Chapter 22 discusses in more detail, disaster planners utilize additional means to accomplish the final step of process improvement described in the preparedness cycle. This final step of the preparedness cycle (i.e., the "I" of "OTEI") serves as a critical connection point between the mission area plan and whatever cycle of process improvement is applied [e.g., Deming's TQM™ or Six Sigma's™ Define. Measure, Analyze, Improve, Control (DMAIC)].

18.5 Case Study: Creating an EOP for Pyronesia

The Pyronesia Ministry of Health has received a Presidential mandate to create an EOP based upon hazards identified in their National Risk Assessment (see Tables 17.1 and 18.2).

Table 18.2 represents a capability inventory that identified thirty core public health capabilities related to emergency response in Pyronesia.

In this case study, Pyronesian EOP stakeholders drafted strategic goals and operational objectives for water, sanitation, and hygiene. Table 18.3 is an example of the SOARR™ planning format used to draft the EOP for the strategic objective of water, sanitation, and hygiene (WASH) (see also Table 13.4).

Table 18.2. Thirty core emergency response capabilities affecting public health in Pyronesia

1. Disease prevention and control
2. Emergency operations coordination
3. Fatality management / mortuary care
4. Food safety, food security, and nutrition
5. Hazmat emergency response / decontamination
6. Health services
7. Health system and infrastructure support
8. Information sharing
9. Injury prevention and control
10. Mass care / shelter & settlement
11. Medical surge
12. Mental health services
13. Nonpharmaceutical interventions (PPE, social distancing, travel restriction/advisory)
14. Occupational health & safety
15. Pest and vector control
16. Population protection measures (evacuation/shelter in place)
17. Public health surveillance / epidemiological investigation
18. Public health laboratory testing
19. Reproductive health services
20. Resource management
21. Responder safety and health
22. Risk assessment and exposure modeling
23. Risk communication / public information and warning
24. Sanitation, excreta disposal, and hygiene promotion
25. Security
26. Situational awareness
27. Social services
28. Solid waste management
29. Volunteer management
30. Water, sanitation, and hygiene

18.6 Case Study: Creating a Preparedness Plan for Pyronesia

After developing the EOP, Pyronesian planners then created a preparedness plan based upon gaps noted during the intervening capacity gap analysis (see Chapter 19). One of the gaps identified involved the following WASH-related activity, "Ensure that the average water available for drinking, cooking, and personal hygiene in any household is at least fifteen liters per person per day." At present, Pyronesia can deliver fifteen liters per person per day to only 1,000 persons. This measurement represents the current capacity ($C_{current}$). Impact analyses identified several high probability hazards that could displace 10,000 persons (e.g., floods, hazardous material releases, earthquakes). This measurement represents the predicted capacity ($C_{predicted}$) that the risk assessment has estimated would be necessary for this incident. The preparedness plan is intended to fill the gap between predicted capacity and current capacity.

Table 18.3. Example of the Pyronesia public health EOP for the capability of WASH

Capability	Strategic Objective	Operational Objective	Activity	Responsible Party	Resources
Water, Sanitation, and Hygiene (WASH)	An adequate supply of clean water is accessible to all people.	A sufficient quantity of water is available to all people.	Ensure that the maximum distance from any household to the nearest water point is 500 meters. Ensure that the average water available for drinking, cooking, and personal hygiene in any household is at least fifteen liters per person per day.	Public works	Staffing Time Equipment Transportation Communications
		Water is of sufficient quality to be potable and used for hygiene.	Ensure there is low risk of fecal contamination. Use a sanitary survey to indicate the risk of fecal contamination. Ensure there are no fecal coliforms per 100 ml at the point of delivery.	Public health	Staffing Time Testing equipment Survey tool Transportation Communications
		People are able to safely collect, store, and use sufficient quantities of water.	Ensure each household has at least two clean water collecting containers of ten-to-twenty liters Ensure water collection and storage containers have narrow necks and/or covers (or other safe means of storage, drawing, and handling).	Military	Staffing Time Containers Transportation Communications

The preparedness plan does so by way of organizing, equipping, and training the responsible parties to perform each activity named in the EOP; and then using process improvement techniques (e.g., Deming's PDCA cycle™, Six Sigma DMAIC™) to evaluate their performance of the activity during an exercise or simulation. After-action studies of these activities provide a list of **corrective actions** for plan improvement, and then the cycle is repeated.

18.7 Questions for Discussion

1. Describe how the preparedness cycle is based upon a hybrid version of the Deming cycle (Plan–Do–Check–Act) for quality control and Fayol's five functions of management (e.g., planning, organizing, staffing, leading, and controlling).
2. Preparedness has been called a polysemous concept. Describe why it is vital to base preparedness activities directly upon *measurable* gaps in the EOP activities.
3. Renowned CDC disaster scientist Dr. Erik Auf der Heide has said that "Disaster plans are an illusion of preparation unless accompanied by training." Describe the significance of this observation as it relates to the role of a preparedness plan.

Chapter

19

Gap Analysis

19.1 Learning Objectives

Upon completion of the chapter, the reader can:

1. Define the following phrase:
   - Surge capacity.

2. Compare and contrast capability and capacity.
3. Describe capacity as a rate-limiting step for emergency operations.

19.2 Checking Planning Assumptions

As depicted in Figure 19.1, the next phase of the planning wheel after creating an emergency operations plan (EOP) is to compare that EOP to the previously developed planning assumptions in search of any gaps that may be remediated through preparedness.

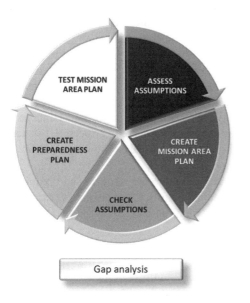

Figure 19.1 Gap analysis as a step in the third phase of the planning wheel

Recall from Chapter 3 that capacity is defined as "the combination of all the strengths, attributes, and resources available that can be used to achieve agreed goals." Capacity is typically expressed as a rate (e.g., #kcal food/day, #liters/water/person/day, #patients treated/day).

The capacity analysis goal is to measure (or estimate) capacity, the maximum rate at which stakeholders can perform a capability. This information about capacity is then used to perform a gap analysis – comparing the EOP with the planning assumptions.

For example, one of the core capabilities identified during the capability inventory for Pyronesia was health services. The capacity of healthcare services varies according to different specialties. While Pyronesia has the *capability* to provide medical care for both adults and children, the *capacity* to treat children is much lower than that for adults. This capacity has measurable indicators (i.e., pediatric hospital bed capacity, the number of pediatricians).

19.3 Defining Capacity

In the past, capacity has been rather narrowly defined as "the combination of all the strengths, attributes, and resources available in a community, society, or organization that can be used to minimize (adverse outcomes) *following* exposure to a hazard" [74, p. 6].

However, contrary to this somewhat dated definition, capacity is not only applied following hazard exposure (i.e., during response and recovery) and *beforehand* to reduce or eliminate risk (i.e., during prevention, protection, and mitigation). Like preparedness, stakeholders routinely apply capacity in all mission areas to prevent, protect themselves from, mitigate the impacts of, respond to, and recover from disasters.

Populations apply individual, household, community, and societal capacity [35]. This capacity includes economic, material, behavioral, and sociopolitical resources for reducing the risk of disaster-related health outcomes

Capacity is often erroneously represented only as an asset inventory (i.e., number of meals, amount of water, number of tents). However, this application recognizes only resources. It does not consider the efficiency of operations that implement capacity and effectively increase the outcome's certainty. In other words, the mere existence of a capacity does not ensure its maximum utilization over time. On the contrary, (as any experienced emergency manager can tell you), the efficient utilization of capacity is notoriously tricky during emergency response operations.

Capacity may also be considered as an input to the system that influences the rate of outcomes. It reflects the rate at which a system can deliver (i.e., functionality) and not merely the available inventory. Therefore, capacity is measured as a performance rate over time (i.e., number of meals delivered per day; liters of water delivered per person, per day; the number of tents erected per day). Thus, the maximum capacity (not the resources) represents a rate-limiting step for reducing disaster impact [35].

EOPs are intended to assist populations in maximizing limited resources and reducing disaster-related health outcomes. Capacity assessments identify those resources (e.g., core capabilities with corresponding capacities) that are required to reduce the incidence of disease for each of the hazards.

Components of "resilience capacity" applied to risk acceptance/retention (i.e., response and recovery) include absorptive, adaptive, and transformative capacities [35]. These three elements commonly vary along a continuum. This continuum is related to the level of change necessary for recovery and the transactional cost associated with doing so.

On one end of the spectrum is absorptive capacity, the measure of an ability to absorb and assimilate the effects of hazard exposure. Absorptive capacity is based upon the system's stability and its function to buffer impact without significant change in the process itself. Adaptive capacity requires less stability and more flexibility to make incremental adjustments in the process to improve. And finally, transformative capacity is a measure of the ability to transform or change processes entirely to optimize outcomes. Transformative capacity requires the highest degree of system flexibility and comes at the highest transactional cost [35]

Individuals, households, communities, and societies each tend to apply these three capacity elements in nearly sequential order during a response. Initially, those systems affected respond by rapidly absorbing inputs (i.e., patients, displaced people) to a given threshold (i.e., **surge capacity**), then adapting to accommodate a larger, more efficient, or more effective version of the same process (e.g., coordination with local emergency response),and then finally the transformation of the entire process into one that is more suitable for the expected outcome (i.e., multinational humanitarian assistance).

19.4 The Capacity Gap ($C_{current} - C_{predicted}$)

The gap analysis is intended to identify gaps in capacity that constrain or hinder emergency response operations' effectiveness. During the risk assessment, stakeholders perform a hazard characterization that provides actionable intelligence for estimating what capabilities are needed. Then, during subsequent plan-writing, stakeholders elaborate upon these capabilities to describe activities and resources to ensure their successful completion.

This step is accomplished first by writing an EOP based upon current capabilities and capacity. A gap analysis is then performed to compare current levels of capability to those predicted by the risk assessment. Somewhat counterintuitive to the timing of its implementation, the preparedness plan is created after the EOP, not beforehand.

Thus, the EOP provides a detailed estimate of the capacities associated with each capability (usually in terms of resources like personnel, materials, and time). Rates may be then estimated for all activities in the plan, and the productivity rates are calculated for plan outputs (e.g., number of household surveys completed/worker/day; or number of meals delivered/worker/hour).

These rates are represented as current and predicted response capacity. The maximum *current* response capacity ($C_{current}$) is estimated as the maximum delivery rate for a capability identified in the EOP. Maximum *predicted* response capacities ($C_{predicted}$) are then estimated using data regarding needs predicted by the risk assessment (e.g., number of injured, the number killed, number displaced). The current capacity is then compared to the expected capacity, and gaps are noted. These gaps are then remediated using a preparedness plan as the guide. The result is a preparedness plan that is focused and prioritized to address the most critical needs using our core capabilities.

This entire process is summarized as follows:

1. Capability inventory

   - Identify those capabilities that are required to reduce disease incidence.

2. Risk assessment

   - Estimate the predicted capacity ($C_{predicted}$) needed for this capability.

3. Create an EOP
   - Identify response activities and resources.
4. Gap analysis
   - Estimate the current capacity ($C_{current}$) held for each capability in the EOP.
   - Calculate the gap between the current capacity and expected capacity to improve disaster-related health outcomes.
5. Create a preparedness plan
   - Identify preparedness activities and resources.

19.5 Case Study: Performing a Gap Analysis for Hospital Surge Capacity in Pyronesia

As part of its Presidential mandate for planning, the Pyronesia Ministry of Health performed a gap analysis of capability #6 in their capability inventory, health services (see Table 18.2).

In this case study, Pyronesian planners are working with the national healthcare providers to perform a capacity gap analysis of healthcare system capabilities (i.e., primary, secondary, and tertiary care).

Table 19.1 provides a listing of predicted disaster impacts on the hospital system for select disaster hazards in Pyronesia.

Table 19.2 compares current capacities for healthcare to those capacities predicted to become needed during an epidemic.

As indicated in Table 19.2, the capacity gap analysis for health services in Pyronesia has revealed a likely and potentially huge gap in mortuary services, emergency medical and outpatient services, and laboratory testing that would be needed during a human epidemic.

Table 19.1. Predicted impacts of select disaster hazards on the healthcare system of Pyronesia

	Human epidemic	Severe storms	Road crash
Deaths	4,000	4	20
Notifiable illnesses	200,000	0	0
Hospitalizations	2,0000	100	100
Accident and emergency department visits	100,000	200	250
Outpatient visits	150,000	400	50
Surgeries	0	25	50
X-rays	10,000	50	100
CT and MRI scans	0	5	10
Laboratory tests	10,000	50	100
Ambulance runs	5,000	50	50

Table 19.2. Capacity gap analysis for the Pyronesia healthcare system capability

Medical capability	Routine weekly capacity	30 percent surge capacity	Maximum weekly capacity, $C_{Current}$	Weekly $C_{Predicted}$ for epidemic	Weekly capacity gap for epidemic
Mortuary services	83	25	108	4,000 ± 1,000	−3,892 ± 1,000
Notifiable illnesses	29	9	28	200,000 ± 20,000	N/A
Hospitalizations	3,914	1174	5,088	5,0000 ± 1,000	+88
Accident and emergency visits	27,590	8,227	35,867	100,000 ± 10,000	−64,133 ± 10,000
Outpatient visits	17,057	5,252	22,759	150,000 ± 25,0000	−127,241 ± 25,000
Surgeries	809	243	1,052	0	+1,052
X-rays	10,048	3,014	13,062	10,000 ± 1,000	+3,062
CT and MRI scans	220	66	286	100 ± 10	+186
Laboratory tests	149,408	44,822	194,230	200,000 ± 20,000	−5,770 ± 20,000
Ambulance runs	454	136	590	5,000 ± 1,000	−4,410 ± 1,000

The preparedness plan is intended to identify and employ means that build additional capacity. For example, this additional capacity may include adaptive capacity, supplemented by adaptation of treatment settings, to include outpatient drive-throughs that could increase patient throughput. And finally, transformative capacity may also be added by transforming the response into a multinational humanitarian assistance effort.

19.6 Questions for Discussion

1. The daily recommended requirement for water is fifteen liters/person/day. Describe the ability to deliver water at a rate of one liter/person/day, in terms of current capacity and predicted capacity.
2. Draft a (SMART) preparedness plan objective that describes how this water gap will be addressed.

Chapter

Plan Implementation

20

20.1 Learning Objectives

Upon completion of the chapter, the reader can:

1. Define the following terms and phrases:
   - Common operating picture
   - Echelon
   - Essential elements of information
   - Information exchange
   - Operational intelligence
   - Situational awareness
   - Unified command.

2. Describe the flow of information between the EOC and a field command post regarding the incident action plan and the EOP.
3. List the five phases of incident action planning.
4. List the three goals of information exchange.
5. Define deliberate planning.

20.2 Incident Management

As discussed in Chapter 17, risk represents future events that have not yet occurred. Once an event occurs, it is referred to as an "incident." Effective incident management helps to ensure that all stakeholders' efforts are coordinated and synchronized to achieve the best results. Therefore, organizations create incident action plans (IAPs) that guide the implementation of the emergency operations plan (EOP) within an incident command system (ICS). IAPs serve to assign an operational period for implementation of the EOP. This operational period allows the various stakeholders to synchronize operations at the incident level and assure that incident operations are conducted supporting the EOP. This synchronization requires an efficient system for the exchange of information.

Figure 20.1 depicts how IAPs facilitate the coordination between multiple field incident sites (i.e., field command posts) and the centrally coordinated emergency operations center (EOC). Within this **unified command** structure, the IAPs implemented by the field command posts are intended to execute the EOP as managed by the EOC. All strategic goals and operational objectives should be the same for both **echelons**. Activities may vary

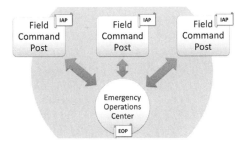

Figure 20.1 Information flow between EOC and field command posts during a disaster

somewhat according to the specific event. These IAP variances from the EOP are reconciled between the field command posts and the EOC.

20.3 Information Exchange

In addition to an organizational structure, the ICS also serves as a system for information exchange.

The EOP and the IAPs form the logical framework for the exchange of **operational intelligence**.

The three goals of this information exchange relate to **situational awareness** (SA), a **common operating picture** (COP), and to ensure the availability of **essential elements of information** (EEI). (See Chapter 21 for a detailed discussion of **information exchange**.)

20.4 Incident Action Planning

Incident action planning is the vehicle by which EOP stakeholders communicate their expectations regarding the execution of the EOP. IAPs provide additional guidance regarding the operational and tactical details of incident response. For EOCs (representing all EOP stakeholders) to communicate these expectations to field command posts, EOPs must first communicate with IAPs.

As discussed in Chapter 13, the SOARR™ format represents a "hierarchy of hypotheses" that is well suited for a hierarchy of plans. IAPs are compliant with the operational objectives identified in EOPs. And, in turn, EOPs are compliant with national goals and plans. (e.g., the national response plan). This hierarchy (i.e., planning assumptions, strategic, operational, and tactical plans) is also well suited for the delegation of authority and scalability within an ICS.

Figure 20.2 illustrates the so-called planning p for incident action planning. Note that (like the planning cycle), "the planning p" also represents a modified version of Deming's cycle (see Figure 1.1). In other words, the "planning p" is an iterative quality control loop applied to incident action planning.

As illustrated in Figure 20.2, the "planning p" represents the five phases of incident action planning as follows:

1. understand the situation,
2. establish incident objectives,
3. develop the IAP,
4. prepare and disseminate the IAP, and
5. execute, evaluate, and revise the IAP.

The IAP identifies incident objectives and provides essential information regarding the incident organization, resource allocation, work assignments, safety, and weather [4, 87].

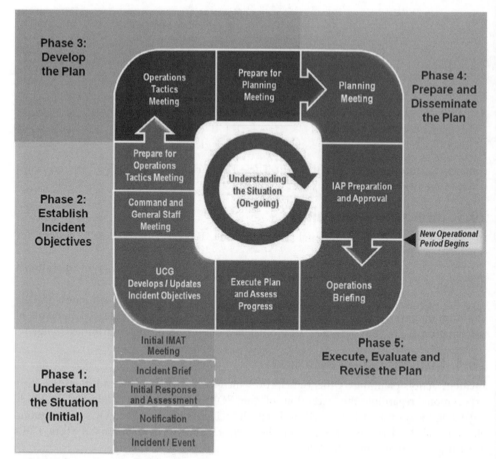

Figure 20.2 The "planning p" for incident action planning.
Source: FEMA [4]
Permission: Non-proprietary government publication

20.5 Understanding the Situation

The first phase of incident action planning involves situational awareness. Initially, this includes an emergency notification of the event, initial response and assessment, and a series of preliminary informational meetings. This situational awareness aims to collect data regarding the operating environment, comprehend the significance of the situation, and *predict* future events and outcomes [87]. (See Chapter 21 for a more detailed discussion of situational awareness.) This information typically includes both EEIs and specific EEIs requested by incident managers, known as critical information requests (CIR).

20.6 Establish Incident Objectives

At the beginning of an incident, the situation is chaotic and situational awareness is difficult to obtain. Therefore, the needs of the affected population are rarely accurately assessed within the first 24 hours of a major national disaster, and actions must therefore be based upon **deliberate planning**. Deliberate planning encompasses the preparation of plans in non-crisis situations (as compared to incident planning, which occurs after a crisis) [88]. Deliberate plans are used to develop contingencies for a broad range of activities based on planning directives' requirements. EOPs represent a form of deliberate planning and may be used to determine priorities and objectives for the initial IAP when situational awareness and other sources of information are limited. After that, the IAP should continue to reference and adapt the objectives and tasks in the EOP.

20.7 Develop the IAP

National and regional support becomes integrated with local incident management through incident action planning. IAPs begin with the operational objectives and related activities of the EOP. In essence, the activities of the EOP are translated to become the operational objectives of the IAP – each with its cascading subset of incident-specific activities, responsible parties, and resources. The field incident manager is responsible for assigning resources according to the responsible parties named in the EOP. The field command post-ICS is then responsible for coordinating review and alterations of the EOP with the EOC to inform subsequent IAP development for each operational period (usually daily). Unresolved conflicts between the EOP and IAP are typically resolved, as needed among incident managers and key stakeholders.

The ICS operations section typically matches the work required to execute the tactics using resources to create individual work assignments. As work assignments are developed, the ICS safety officer, logistics section chief, and the security manager typically review the work assignments and provide input.

20.8 Prepare and Disseminate the IAP

The ICS planning section is usually responsible for preparing, gaining approval of, and disseminating the IAP. In the United States, the IAP process involves completing multiple forms as part of a standardized system for IAP documentation. Among these forms is an operational planning worksheet that assists the ICS operations section in documenting tactics and identifying resources. The SOARR™ planning format may also be used to create these same IAPs with practical planning principles consistently (e.g., O2C3). The resultant standardized IAPs may also be disseminated according to the same means as the EOP, including the same digital platforms.

20.9 Execute, Evaluate, and Revise the IAP

The IAP is intended to be executed and evaluated during each operational period (usually for every eight-hour shift or daily). Each operational period should begin with an operational briefing to discuss the IAP for the upcoming operational period.

Monitoring and evaluating the work's efficiency and effectiveness during each operational period is essential to drive activities for the following operational period. Examples of these measures may include the following indicators: the extent to which objectives were achieved, the rate at which resources were depleted, predicted resource shortfalls and surpluses for the next operational period, and significant changes in dynamic conditions such as weather and security.

Ideally, these critical measures of response performance are available through digital information exchange systems that allow for data aggregation and operational presentations for manager access (e.g., a data dashboard).

20.10 Mass Casualty Incident in Pyronesia

A mass casualty incident has occurred in Pyronesia. There are initial reports of a train derailment that occurred within a densely populated area near the capitol. The Pyronesia National Emergency Management Office (PYRO-NEMO) has activated its EOC. The Pyronesia Ministry of Health has been identified as the lead support agency and is also present at the EOC.

Two field command posts have been activated, one at the scene of the incident (with a fire chief serving as the incident commander) and a second at the nation's largest (and closest) trauma center, Dever National Hospital located in Caldera. Both command posts have already activated their respective disaster plans, have notified staff, and have begun to establish emergency operations. Both the hospital and the on-scene command post have cellular telephone and Wi-Fi internet access.

At the National EOC, the ministry of health planners begin to work with the planning sections of the two command posts to ensure hospital and field staff access to the national EOP, including the capabilities of "health services" and "medical surge." Using the EOP, both peripheral command posts establish an initial set of critical objectives (that guide the initial field IAP response and the subsequent hospital EOP response) and draft a corresponding set of critical information requirements (that guide the national EOP response).

After implementing the first set of objectives within an eight-hour operational period, the IAP planning section is then able to review and revise EOP activities to accommodate the specific needs of the situation. Meanwhile, the EOC is working to coordinate with the Pyronesia military, and police response plans to add security and traffic control capabilities along with the Service d'Aide Médicale Urgente (Urgent Medical Aid Service) (SAMU) ambulance system for patient transportation to the hospital. The EOC logistics section has also worked to ensure robust radio and telephone communications are maintained between the EOC, the hospital, the ambulances, the command post, and responders working on the scene. They all refer to a hierarchy of plans including the National EOP, the Hospital EOP, and the on-scene IAP.

20.11 Question for Discussion

The scene's unfolding realities often require a revision of IAP activities to accommodate unforeseen circumstances and uncertainty. This revision may also include EOP operational or even strategic objectives, ideally performed in partnership with the EOC. Describe how unified command is intended to resolve these issues.

Chapter

21

Plan Sharing

21.1 Learning Objectives

Upon completion of the chapter, the reader can:

1. Define the following terms and phrases:
   - Artificial intelligence
   - B-tree
   - Cognition
   - Data component
   - Data sharing
   - Data structure
   - Database language
   - Evidence-based decision-making
   - Extensible Markup Language (XML)
   - Feedback loop
   - Information
   - Information sharing
   - Intelligence
   - Judgment
   - Knowledge
   - Operational intelligence
   - Peer-to-peer networks
   - Prediction
   - Processing
   - Structured Query Language (SQL)
   - Understanding.
2. Compare and contrast the B-tree self-balancing data structure to the hierarchical data structure of the ADEPT™ system.
3. Describe why it is essential to use a standard data language for disaster-related information sharing.
4. Describe how the ADEPT™ system applies principles of operational intelligence to query an emergency operations plan.
5. Describe the hierarchy of operational intelligence in terms of data, information, knowledge, understanding, and intelligence.
6. Describe the feedback loop for learning that exists between information and knowledge.
7. List the three goals of emergency information exchange.

8. List Endsley's three levels of situational awareness.
9. List the three facets of situational awareness.
10. Describe why response staff typically receive only essential elements of information, rather than the entire common operating picture.

21.2 Data for Decision-Making

Data is a set of facts, measurements, and observations collected for reference or analysis. A database is an organized collection of data, generally stored and accessed electronically from a computer system. When data is processed, organized, structured, or presented within a given context to make it useful, it is called information. This data for decision-making can be used to inform future courses of action.

The scientific method is then used to test the relationships that exist within the data. The resulting evidence is then interpreted to become new knowledge. When we create this new knowledge, it influences our ability to understand other information (i.e., evidence). Evidence-based decision-making is the process used for making decisions grounded in the best available evidence (i.e., research, experiential, and contextual). By using evidence-based decision-making, emergency managers can minimize uncertainty and variability during the accomplishment of plan objectives.

21.3 Organizing Electronic Data

Computer software applications are comprised of two main components: language and data. A set of standardized languages is used to create instructions for how the software operates and how the electronic data is managed.

The specific format used for organizing, managing, and storing data is called a **data structure**. A data structure includes **data components**, the relationships among them, and the functions applied to the data. It is related to the formal data names, comprehensive data definitions, and precise data integrity rules. Data structures enable efficient access and modification of the database and allow for quick queries and functional manipulations of the data. A data structure manifests a specific data schema for a specific purpose within an organization's data resource.

A **B-tree** is a type of self-balancing tree data structure that maintains sorted data and allows searches, sequential access, insertions, and deletions in logarithmic time. It is particularly well suited for storage systems that read and write relatively large blocks of data, such as disks, and is commonly used in databases and file systems.

"Music is given to us with the sole purpose of *establishing an order in things,* including, and particularly, the coordination between man and time"

– Igor Stravinsky

A database schema is a diagrammatic representation of the data structure. Out of context, descriptions within the individual data units (e.g., specific plan goals, objectives, activities, and responsible parties) do little to inform the overall process. However, (like the notes of a song) when these individual data units are combined in a specific order, they deliver a logical message. This specific order for organizing the data is referred to as a database schema. This schema refers to the organization of data like a blueprint depicting how the database is constructed. In a relational database, the schema defines the tables, fields, relationships, views, and other elements. Database schema may be considered as the logical framework of the entire database.

21.4 Managing Electronic Data

These relationships among the data are described using a common **database language**, a class of languages used to define and manage databases. A query language is a computer language used to make queries in databases and information systems. Many relational database systems use **Structured Query Language** (SQL) for querying and maintaining the database. However, SQL implementations can be incompatible among some software applications and do not necessarily follow standards.

Extensible Markup Language (XML) is a markup language that defines rules for encoding documents using tags to define the various elements for later retrieval. Although the design of XML focuses on documents, XML is now widely used for communicating data between database applications, especially those used in web services. XML has also been proposed as a national standard language used for sharing disaster-related information [89]. The ADEPT™ database approach has been translated into multiple languages, including XML (which also allowed for the highest degree of functionality compared to other languages).

The National Information Exchange Model (NIEM) is an XML-based information exchange framework used in the United States. NIEM is used across all government levels (i.e., local, state, tribal, territorial, and federal). It is designed to support enterprise-wide information exchange standards and processes throughout multiple governmental sectors (e.g., justice, public safety, emergency and disaster management, intelligence, and homeland security [89].

Intelligence is the actionable insight necessary for evidence-based decision-making.

21.5 Integrating Data into Decision-Making

Operational intelligence is an event-centric approach to integrating information that allows managers to make better decisions based on evidence [90]. Operational intelligence applications typically run data queries to deliver analytic results in the form of operational instructions [91].

The word **intelligence** is a polysemous term. In the broadest sense (and in the case of education), intelligence is intended to describe the ability to apply knowledge to understand better and predict future events. When applied more precisely (e.g., national defense), intelligence describes the ability to apply knowledge to understand and predict future threats. In all cases, intelligence is based upon an understanding that allows for decisions that improve predictability and lessen variability among future outcomes. Intelligence results from a series of procedures that refine data into actionable items used in predictive modeling for future outcomes. These procedures include **processing, cognition, judgment**, and **prediction** (see Figure 21.1) [92].

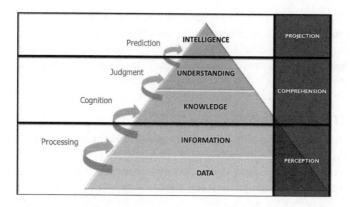

Figure 21.1 Hierarchy of operational intelligence, according to three levels of situational awareness

As illustrated in Figure 21.1, processing refines data to create information. Thus, data is an individual unit that contains a raw material that does not carry any specific meaning. Information is a group of data that collectively carry a logical meaning. The information represents data that has been processed to be relevant for the end-user.

Cognition is the process of acquiring knowledge using thought, experience, and the senses. Cognition allows us to comprehend **information** and convert it into **knowledge**. A positive **feedback loop** also exists between information and knowledge. Insights gained from the interpretation of information leads to new knowledge – a new actionable "rule" that can then, in turn, be applied to other information. We commonly call this feedback loop "learning." It is also critical to developing machine learning as a basis for **artificial intelligence**.

Judgment is the ability to make decisions and draw conclusions. **Understanding** occurs when we perceive the significance, explanation, or cause of something. Judgment refines knowledge to create understanding. For example, experienced emergency managers use their judgment to complement their knowledge, resulting in a deeper understanding of an incident's causes and significance.

Prediction is the ability to forecast the nature of a future event. This forecasting allows for the planning and projection of additional capabilities that would not otherwise be available at the last minute. The predictability of future operations improves the variability of performance and certainty of outcomes. Intelligence allows for an evidence-based prediction of an intended future goal (e.g., statistical probability) along with an associated measure of uncertainty (e.g., statistical confidence).

Operational intelligence is a category of real-time dynamic, business analytics that delivers insight into data, events, and operations. Solutions run queries against streaming data feeds and event data to deliver analytic results. This insight provides organizations the ability to make decisions and immediately act on these analytic insights through manual or automated actions. Just as data informs information to create knowledge, knowledge then, in turn, informs understanding that results in actionable intelligence. Operational intelligence is intended to guide this process of evidence-based decision-making.

21.6 Exchanging Electronic Information

Information exchange (i.e., **information sharing**) describes data exchange between various people, organizations, and technologies [93]. There are three types of information sharing:

(1) information shared by individuals, (2) information shared by organizations, and (3) information shared by software.

Information sharing differs from **data sharing**. In information sharing, the data is already processed, organized, structured, or presented within a given context before it is shared. In comparison, data sharing typically involves sharing access to raw data in the form of a database or a collection of individual data units.

In the past, traditional information sharing referred to one-to-one exchanges between a sender and receiver; or messages broadcasted from one sender to many receivers. With the advent of modern **peer-to-peer networks**, it is now possible to share information in both directions – from many-to-one and many-to-many [94].

Table 21.1 compares these two architectures' various characteristics and the implications for each social system during a disaster response.

Among other functionality, this also allows for more effective communication of ideas between any number of senders and receivers. It also provides a feedback loop for testing communication effectiveness, including public information and risk communication.

Rarely do modern emergency operations receive too little information. It is now much more common to be overwhelmed by too much information. For this reason, it is necessary to manage the exchange of information according to the specific needs of the end-user.

> "The absorptive capacity of responders is pretty low. It's not because they do not have an affinity to technology. It's because they are really, really busy 98% of the time, and they are sleeping the other 2%"
>
> – Robert Kirkpatrick, United Nations Global Pulse

The goals of emergency information exchange are three-fold: (1) to maintain situational awareness (SA) regarding the incident, (2) to provide a common operating picture (COP) for planning and implementing "smart" strategic goals and operational objectives, and

Table 21.1. A comparison of key characteristics of peer-to-peer and hierarchical architecture

	Peer-to-Peer	Hierarchical
Users	Public	Institutions
Sanction	Non-official	Official
Empowerment	Individual	Organizational
Activation	Immediate	Delayed
Adaptability	High	Moderate
Accessibility	Inclusive	Exclusive
Sources of public information	Many	One
Structure	Dynamic	Static
Scalability	High	Moderate

Source: From Keim and Noji, AJDM [94]
Permission: Purchased from AJDM on January 14, 2021

(3) to ensure that essential elements of information (EEI) are available for accomplishment of response activities by the appropriate responsible party.

21.7 Situational Awareness

Endsley's model of situational awareness includes the following three levels: (1) *perception* – of the operating environment (i.e., access to data and orientation to time and space); (2) *comprehension* – of the significance of the situation; and (3) *projection* of the situation onto future states and events [87] (see also Figure 21.1).

For example, an on-scene incident commander at a train derailment fire may *perceive* the risk of a particularly dangerous (but hidden) explosive phenomenon related to boiling liquids inside the pressurized tank cars. These boiling-liquid, expanding-vapor explosions (i.e., BLEVEs) characteristically result in enormous explosions. An emergency manager's technical knowledge, along with data from the train manifest, allows them to *comprehend* the likelihood of increased risk over time in the area closest to the pressurized cars. They can then *project* the potential impact of such an enormous explosion (e.g., blast and plume modeling) and take measures to protect responders and the public (e.g., scene safety and population evacuation).

> "It is important to distinguish the term situation awareness, as a state of knowledge, from the processes used to achieve that state"
>
> – Mica Endsley

There are three facets of SA as follows: states, systems, and processes. States refer to the actual awareness of the situation. Systems refer to the exchange of information between parts. Processes refer to the ongoing actions of updating during a rapid change of events.

Within this context, situational awareness is a measurable outcome. In other words, situational awareness may be considered as a core capability of emergency response. Emergency operations typically perform operational-level situation assessments that inform strategic-level situation awareness. This analysis's long-term strategic goal is typically directed toward projection – prediction of future events or outcomes.

21.8 Common Operating Picture

In the case of SA, the flow of information is managed according to the end-user's specific needs. Emergency managers seek to share a common understanding of the current situation. This common operational picture (COP) is treated as a "single source of truth" that offers comprehensive situational awareness for strategic decision-making [95]. However, downstream assets (i.e., response staff) typically receive only the information that is necessary to help them execute their specific activities (e.g., essential elements of information (EEI) [95]. Figure 21.2 illustrates the relationship between situational awareness, common operating picture, and essential elements of information. For responders, situational awareness is limited to EEIs. For emergency managers, situational awareness also includes information related to the COP, in addition to the EEIs.

21.9 Essential Elements of Information

EEI is information that is essential to accomplish an activity. The EEI is specific to a particular activity and the party (or parties) responsible for completing that activity. The

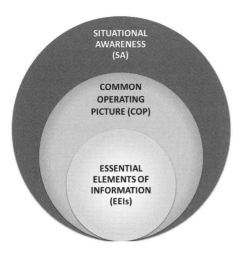

Figure 21.2 Span of information-sharing for situational awareness, common operating picture, and essential elements of information

most effective EEI are written out in advance by end-users of the information (i.e., responsible parties identified in the disaster plan). This accuracy imparted by end-users is another reason why the ADEPT™ planning system always includes the end-users of EEI (i.e., responsible parties identified in the emergency operations plan) in the plan-writing process, along with managers and leaders.

For example, during a disaster, emergency managers for hospital command centers may rapidly require the following EEIs:

- Cause, scale, and scope of the incident.
- Types, numbers, and demographics of casualties.
- Estimated time of arrival.
- Casualty triage categories (i.e., severity).
- Status of the current response.
- Hazardous materials involved (e.g., biologicals, chemicals, radiation).
- Health and safety risk for staff or patients.
- Anticipated medical needs.
- Impact on service delivery.
- Means of communication with incident command.
- Status of the facility, staffing, and supplies.
- Availability of resources, including external aid.

In comparison, Table 21.2 provides another example of twenty-one essential elements of information that are commonly reported during a public health emergency response.

These essential information elements are frequently requested by public health and medical leaders at the national, state, and local levels. These entities commonly request this information to be reported by hospitals, long-term care facilities, community health centers, healthcare coalitions, local public health entities, and health-related nongovernmental organizations (e.g., Red Cross / Red Crescent). Therefore, public health planners should include information sharing as a core capability in their emergency operations plans.

Table 21.2. Essential elements of information commonly identified during a public health emergency response [92–94]

- Location, needs, and demographics of affected population
- Facility operating status and structural integrity
- Status of community evacuations/shelter in-place operations
- Status of critical medical services (e.g., emergency department, trauma, critical care)
- Hospital admissions and bed status
- Critical service/infrastructure status (e.g., electric, water, sanitation, heating, ventilation, and air conditioning)
- Equipment/supplies/medications/vaccine status or needs
- Healthcare staffing
- Patient tracking and evacuation
- Public health staffing and surge capacity
- Electronic medical records
- Coordination of community response
- Emergency Medical Services (EMS) status
- Epidemiological or lab data (e.g., test results, case counts, deaths)
- School-related data (e.g., closure, absenteeism, etc.)
- Points of distribution / mass vaccination sites data (e.g., throughput, set-up status, etc.)
- Diagnostic criteria and case definitions
- Therapeutic regimens
- Clinical trial data
- Genomic data
- Case reports
- Summary results derived from multiple data sources

21.10 Information Sharing among Public Health Agencies

The recent Ebola outbreaks and coronavirus pandemic have raised important issues around rapidly sharing data and results during public health emergencies. According to the World Health Organization (WHO), multiple barriers to rapid information sharing still exist. These barriers relate to the balance of (sometimes competing) priorities associated with information exchange as follows:

- data sharing versus confidentiality,
- rapidity versus accuracy,
- politics versus public health,
- reciprocity versus reporting,
- curation versus collection,
- research versus operations, and
- publication versus dissemination.

While there is no single clear, immediate solution, improving information exchange requires concrete initiatives and resources alongside culture change. WHO has identified multiple opportunities for overcoming these barriers [96]. These opportunities to improve information sharing during public health emergencies included the following:

- regulatory frameworks,
- data sharing platforms for curation, synthesis, and dissemination,
- improvements in journal publication,

- academic reward structures, and
- knowledge curation and management systems.

Public health agencies also use information-sharing systems for the exchange of public health information. While a detailed discussion of health information systems is beyond this book's scope, the practice of information exchange is relatively well developed in public health. Health-related data is commonly shared via electronic surveillance systems. Information is widely available via online collections of publications (e.g., US/HHS TRACIE), electronic databases (e.g., CDC National Notifiable Diseases Surveillance System), tools (e.g., CDC Communication Resource Center), resources (e.g., Worldwide Antimalarial Resistance Network, WWARN), and networks (e.g., the Global Influenza Surveillance Network, GISN).

21.11 Sharing Plan Information

One of the defining attributes of the ADEPT™ planning system is using an electronic database to collect, store, and access data from a computer system [13]. This plan data represents the best evidence available for decision-making. The planning assumptions are based upon evidence gained from research, experience, and context. The relative calm of the planning period permits a more deliberative process for considering courses of action based upon the best available evidence for decision-making, not merely our best guess under pressure.

Evidence-informed, iterative, group-based planning allows for data to be extensively refined through collective processing, cognition, judgment, and prediction. The result of this planning effort is an emergency operations plan (EOP) – a collection of intelligence that allows for valid and accurate prediction of future stakeholder activity, according to the best evidence available. This collection exists in multiple degrees of development, ranging from uninterpreted raw data (e.g., resources) to intelligence (e.g., goals and objectives). An application for operational intelligence then operates by querying an ADEPT™ database to deliver results in an instructional (activity-based) format.

The ADEPT™ system involves the use of a set of tables represented as a B-tree self-balancing data structure. This data structure allows for quick queries and functional manipulations of the ADEPT™ hierarchical tree (see Figure 13.1). The ADEPT™ tree parses data into progressively divided branches of strategic goals that unfold as operational objectives, activities, responsible parties, and resources.

The ADEPT™ system also uses a standardized database schema for organizing plan information (i.e., the SOARR™ format) [13, 28]. This SOARR™ hierarchical format serves as a database schema for describing the relationships of the database, where these data are divided into database tables. In other words, the SOARR™ schema serves as the logical framework for the entire database.

These relationships among ADEPT™ system data are easily described using XML, a standard database language used to define and manage databases and designed to support enterprise-wide information exchange standards and processes throughout multiple public and governmental sectors.

The ADEPT™ system applies principles of operational intelligence to query a database for operational instructions. This database is comprised of the EOP represented in electronic format. Queries deliver results in instructions for emergency operations that include plan objectives, activities, and resources. This event-centric approach for integrating evidence and decision-making allows emergency managers to make decisions that improve predictability and lessen variability among future outcomes.

Another characteristic of the ADEPT™ system related to operational intelligence is the use of techniques that allow for refining of data to become actionable intelligence. These analytical techniques are performed within a group forum for iteration among plan stakeholders. Data is further processed into usable information during the planning sessions, as stakeholders acquire knowledge of the content, process it, and then apply their judgment to understand the situation. They then apply a consensus-based model for decision-making to predict future events and capabilities. Expectedly, this process also drives the feedback loop of learning. As stakeholders gain new knowledge, they can recognize patterns in otherwise meaningless information, creating new knowledge. When this occurs during planning, the entire group learns as a result. Thus, the stakeholders themselves are also changed by participation.

> "The highest reward for a man's toil is not what he gets for it, but what he becomes by it"
>
> – John Ruskin

During this planning process, all stakeholders collaborate to develop progressively higher levels of situational awareness by sharing data, experience, and context related to intelligence. Thus, plan stakeholders exchange information to build mutual situational awareness before the event. This process progresses according to Endsley's levels as plan stakeholders convene to accomplish the following: (1) perceive the operating environment, (2) comprehend the significance of disaster risk, and (3) project a plan for managing that risk [87].

The database schema of ADEPT™ (i.e., SOARR™) also facilitates the hierarchy of plans introduced initially in Chapter 1. Strategic goals and operational objectives are the primary concern of the "C-suite" and executive-level decision-makers. Operational objectives typically relate to the responsibility of incident managers and response staff. Accordingly, response staff typically need tactical details associated with staffing and resourcing the activities of the plan.

The SOARR™ database schema addresses this need through compartmentalization and distribution of the plan essential elements of information. No longer must the diverse set of plan stakeholders pour over hundreds of pages of the same narrative to identify their instructions. The ADEPT™ database schema simplifies this correlation of the flow of essential elements of information to the appropriate plan stakeholder. Chief executives and regional coordinators can readily perceive, comprehend, and project the plan upon future events at the strategic level. At the same time, incident managers and staff can also rapidly gain situational awareness according to the operational and tactical requirements detailed in the plan. According to other parameters related to national security, information security, and privacy rights, authentication and authorizations can also be used for access control based on a "need to know."

Finally, the ADEPT™ system for plan sharing also provides the opportunity to gain objective and measurable stakeholder feedback with the goal of effective management (e.g., organizing, staffing, leading, and controlling) in real-time. As stakeholders assess and monitor the progress of emergency operations, they continue to test the evidence and assumptions in their EOP against the reality of a common operating picture that is informed by situational awareness. This electronic system then permits automated monitoring and evaluation as the plan objectives are accomplished, including resource allocation measures (time, people, money). Thus, the system provides a dynamic platform for curation, synthesis, dissemination, and *improving the quality* of an EOP.

21.12 Case Study: Information Sharing among the Global Disaster Community

The Virtual On-Site Operations Coordination Centre (OSOCC) is a part of the Global Disaster Alert and Coordination System (GDACS) under the United Nations Office for Coordination of Humanitarian Affairs (UN OCHA) [97]. The online platform, which has been developing for more than a decade, has become a central portal for information sharing related to disasters. With more than 20,000 registered users within the disaster response community, over the last fifteen years, the system has evolved technically and operationally to provide stakeholders with various levels of information in the immediate relief phase following a disaster event [97].

The Virtual OSOCC has facilitated increased information exchange on a global scale. However, as more information from more sources becomes available, analyzing and utilizing it becomes challenging. According to the UN OSOCC, "the challenge is creating an information infrastructure that is sufficiently flexible to manage the dynamic exchange of information among the participating entities in an inter-organizational system but sufficiently ordered to ensure that the relevant information gets to the responsible parties using a validated format and in time to support effective action" (p. 2). One method for achieving this is through the effective use of information–communication technology platforms [97].

Of course, challenges always remain when it comes to coordination of disaster assistance. While the Virtual OSOCC is widely acclaimed in the disaster relief community, the tool is used by select international organizations and not used by governments of the affected countries. According to UN OSOCC studies, increased information sharing does not necessarily translate into an increase in the relevant information. It is also not surprising to hearin the UN OSOCC report that it serves mainly as a facilitator for collaboration through information sharing rather than an actual platform for collaboration [97].

The international community has also developed a cluster architecture to align organizations' efforts with these organizations' divergent methods and values and minimize the risk of conflict within the humanitarian system and the host nation's government [98].

While the cluster system has solved many of earlier systems' problems, challenges related to information management remain persistent. According to the UN Inter-Agency Standing Committee (IASC), the cluster lead agency ensures information management for each sector cluster. However, the clusters tend to manage information best for their own immediate needs and not necessarily for the overall system's information needs [98]. This resulting information fragmentation remains a common occurrence among nearly all disasters, worldwide. However, this is not a new or isolated occurrence. Unfortunately, most emergency managers remain familiar with the all-too-common euphemisms "siloes of excellence" and "stove-piping" to describe the operational isolation that often accompanies information fragmentation.

21.13 Questions for Discussion

1. Brainstorm for examples of how machine learning could be integrated into the feedback loop between knowledge and information related to a disaster plan.
2. Discuss the following ethical concerns related to information sharing:
   - data sharing versus confidentiality,
   - the rapidity of data collection versus accuracy,
   - political versus public health interests,
   - the burden of reporting versus information reciprocity,
   - information curation versus collection,
   - research versus operational needs, and
   - journal publication versus rapid dissemination.

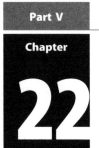

Chapter

22

Plan Monitoring and Evaluation

22.1 Learning Objectives

Upon completion of the chapter, the reader can:

Define the following terms and phrases:

- Common cause variation
- Defect
- Hotwash
- Mass casualty incident (MCI)
- Modeling
- Pareto analysis
- Performance
- Performance indicator
- Performance management
- Performance measure
- Preventive control
- Process control
- Process control analysis
- Process improvement
- Process management
- Process measurement
- Prospective
- Resource management
- Retrospective
- Run charts
- Six Sigma™
- Standard deviation
- Standard error
- Statistical power.

22.2 Operations Management

Chapter 1 described operations as a function of management (and emergency operations as a function of emergency management). Operations management is used to create efficiency within an organization. It is concerned with converting materials and labor into goods (or services) as efficiently as possible to maximize an organization's goals.

Operational planning (e.g., creating an emergency operations plan, EOP) is one of Fayol's five operations management functions that also includes organizing, staffing, leading, and controlling operations. Emergency response operations are then organized, staffed, and led according to the principles of a standardized incident command system (ICS). Controlling is the measuring and correcting of activities to ensure that outcomes conform to plans. In other words, controlling an ICS involves ensuring that incident outcomes conform to the EOP goals and objectives.

Table 1.1 and Figure 1.4 introduced a logic model and framework for public programs in terms of business operations components (i.e., resources, processes, and objectives). Section 7.3 then described operations as a system of inputs, outputs, and outcomes. Table 22.1 describes the relationships between these systems management, business management, the SOARR™ planning format, and key performance measures and indicators (KPIs) for each system component.

Table 22.1. A comparison of operational system components and key performance indicators

System component	Inputs	Outputs	Outcomes
Operational component	Resource	Process	Objective
Management system	Resource management	Process management	Performance management
SOARR™ component	Responsible parties and Resources	Activities	Operational objectives and Strategic goals
Key Performance Indicators (KPIs) and *Performance Measures*	**Resource utilization** • *Time (hours)* • *Staffing (# personnel)* • *Materials (type, amount)* • *Information (EEIs)* **Financing** • *Cost ($USD)*	**Completeness** • *% activities completed* **Efficiency** • *Operational efficiency (activity completed / resource utilized)* • *Productivity* ○ *# activities completed/hour* **Timeliness** • *% of activities with on-time completion* • *Activity cycle time (hours)* **Quality** • *Stakeholder satisfaction (Likert scale)* • *Customer satisfaction (Likert scale)*	**Completeness** • *% goals and objectives completed* **Effectiveness** • *Operational effectiveness (goals and/or objectives completed)* • *Cost- effectiveness ($USD/goal or objective)* **Timeliness** • *% of goals and/or objectives with on-time completion* • *Goal and/or objective cycle time (hours)* **Quality** • *Stakeholder satisfaction (Likert scale)* • *Customer satisfaction (Likert scale)*

22.3 Performance Management

Performance management typically includes two phases: measurement and improvement [10]. Performance measurement is defined as the regular measurement of the outcomes and efficiency of operations. Performance improvement is the practice of using these performance measures to correct problems before they manifest in performance deficiencies [10].

Performance management is based upon the principle of **preventive control**, which assumes that most negative deviations from the plan can be fixed by applying management fundamentals [10]. **Performance** is typically measured and managed during the short-term through monitoring, and during the long-term through evaluation.

22.4 Monitoring and Evaluation

Monitoring is the continuous, **prospective** assessment of ongoing plan activities. It measures progress and helps managers to identify and solve current problems. Monitoring is used to measure the performance of plan activities.

In comparison, an evaluation is a discrete, **retrospective** assessment concerning the relevance, effectiveness, and efficiency of specific objectives. Evaluation is used to measure outcomes and guide future efforts. In other words, monitoring measures the inputs and outputs of activities, and evaluation measures objectives' outcomes. Traditionally, monitoring the implementation of an EOP is performed by the ICS planning section as they create an incident action plan (IAP) in alignment with the EOP or evaluate the existing EOP.

Monitoring includes systems for **resource management** and **process management**. The evaluation includes a system for performance management. Simply stated, resource management is the process by which stakeholders manage their various resources (i.e., inputs) effectively. Process management is the organizational discipline for analyzing, defining, optimizing, monitoring, and controlling processes (i.e., outputs). Finally, performance management is used to define, optimize, monitor, and control the entire operation (i.e., outcomes).

22.5 Process Management

As depicted in Figure 22.1, process management comprises two main phases, process definition and process improvement. This figure also illustrates how the ADEPT™ SOARR™ format connects process definition with process improvement by defining a specific and measurable activity (i.e., process).

Once defined, this process (i.e., activity) may then be improved. Similar to how the SOARR™ format integrates with other well-known process improvement methods (e.g., the preparedness cycle and Deming's PDCA cycle depicted in Figure 18.3), the hierarchical cascade of the ADEPT™ SOARR™ format also integrates well with Six Sigma™. Figure 22.1 illustrates how (like the preparedness cycle in Figure 18.3) the two systems conveniently integrate plan activities – linking process definition with process improvement.

The Six Sigma™ model for process improvement involves defining, measuring, analyzing, improving, and correcting activities to ensure that events conform to plans (DMAIC). Figure 22.1 thus depicts the five steps for improving the efficiency of a process by reducing variability in the process outputs (e.g., process control). In this case, the process has already been well-defined. The specific processes to be improved are the activities of the EOP.

Figure 22.2 illustrates how, during this fifth phase of the planning wheel, stakeholders test the EOP for reliability (reproducibility of the process) and validity (effectiveness of

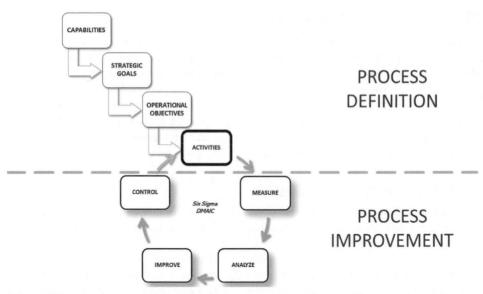

Figure 22.1 Integration of the ADEPT™ SOARR™ format used for process definition with the Six Sigma™ DMAIC model used for process improvement

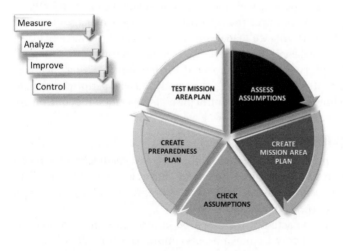

Figure 22.2 Four steps for testing an EOP, as the fifth phase of the planning wheel

outcomes) using these same four steps for testing an EOP (i.e., process improvement) listed as follows (see also Table 14.1):

1. Measure the process (i.e., activity).
2. Analyze the process for variability.
3. Improve the process to reduce variability.
4. Control the process (within an acceptable degree of variability).

22.6 Process Measurement

This chapter discusses the two steps involved with plan monitoring and evaluation (i.e., process measurement and analysis). Chapter 23 discusses the two steps involved with plan quality improvement (i.e., process improvement and control).

As indicated in Figure 22.1, once the activities (i.e., processes) have been defined by plan-writing, the next step of improving the EOP processes begins with assessing the planning assumptions.

Performance measures represent an objective quantification of performance over time. A performance measure should be specific and accurate. It is a numerical expression regarding the extent to which the desired outcome or output has been achieved.

In comparison, performance indicators are indirect qualitative descriptions that require interpretation. **Performance indicators** are a type of performance measurement used to evaluate a particular activity's successful accomplishment according to measurable standards. Key performance indicators (KPIs) compare the observed performance of critical actions to some standard or reference. Performance measures are the means for verifying KPIs.

Table 22.1 lists performance measures that may be applied as indicators of EOP inputs, outputs, and outcomes.

For example, efficiency is a good indicator of process performance. Performance measures for operational efficiency are used as indicators of process efficiency (the number of activities completed per resource utilized) and productivity (the number of activities completed/hour). In comparison, effectiveness is a good indicator of overall operational performance. Performance measures for operational effectiveness include the number of goals and objectives accomplished, as well as cost-effectiveness (number of $USD spent per each outcome)

Process measurement can be better understood by creating process run charts. **Run charts** (also known as run-sequence plots) are simply graphs that display observed data in a time sequence. Run charts are used to depict nonparametric, continuous data. The horizontal x-axis is time, and the vertical y-axis is the process measure of interest. The data is plotted to look for unusual patterns or variations that may represent **defects**.

In service delivery, defects are measured as statistically significant departures from the norm or standard model. These departures are typically reflected by variations in the mean and range of sample values depicted in the process run charts. For example, defects in performance related to completeness may include the number or proportion of EOP activities that remain incomplete at the end of operations or the end of an operational period. Performance defects related to efficiency might involve unusually high levels of resource utilization for accomplishing a given activity. Defects related to timeliness are either related to unusually late completion times or unusually high cycle times. Finally, defects related to quality involve unusually high levels of dissatisfaction expressed by plan users or the people they serve.

22.7 Process Analysis

According to Figure 22.2, the second step in testing the reliability and validity of an EOP is to perform a process analysis (i.e., **process control analysis**) of those performance measures related to each activity in question.

During response operations, incident managers may suspect a high degree of variability in the performance of one activity detailed in the EOP. They may then collect and analyze a sample of data about that activity (e.g., process analysis). This data sample includes multiple trials of the same EOP activity (i.e., process). The total number of trials in the sample is referred to as sample size and is denoted by the letter (n). It is necessary to obtain a sample of at least twelve trials of the same activity (n > 12) to ensure reasonable statistical power. A higher sample size produces more accurate and reproducible (and, therefore, more reliable and valid) results.

22.7.1 Pareto Analysis

This sample is then subjected to quantitative analysis. This statistical analysis begins with a **Pareto analysis** to identify the norm's most frequent defects/variances. It then performs a process control analysis to quantify statistically significant variability in the processes (i.e., EOP activities).

Pareto analyses are typically used to identify the 20 percent of causes that explain 80 percent of the variances measured. It involves the listing of defect types, frequency, and the cost per defect. These values are then used to calculate the total cost of low quality for each defect. This cost is presented as a cumulative percentage of the defects. The resultant graph is used to identify those minority defects (usually 20 percent) responsible for 80 percent of the total cost of low quality (see Figure 22.3).

22.7.2 Process Control Analysis

Once the Pareto analysis has identified defects that are the priority for process improvement, a process control analysis then serves to identify and quantify any process (i.e., EOP activity) that may appear "out of control" (i.e., exhibits a high degree of variability). This analysis begins by creating a simple **run chart** as a quick screening test to see whether the process is in control. In other words, by analyzing the degree to which a process acts as it does typically (with only **common cause variation** and no special cause variation in play). In the next step of process control analysis, process control charts are created. Process control charts are run charts that have been further enhanced to include degrees of standard error represented as upper and lower control limits. Since the standard error is calculated by

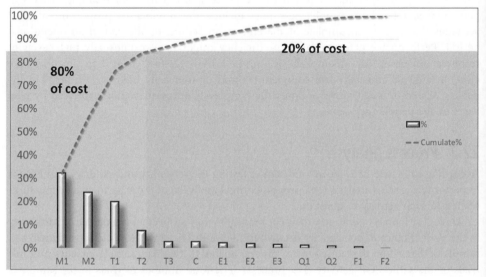

Figure 22.3 Pareto analysis of estimated cost of defects associated with ambulance runs at the national exercise

calculating the standard deviation and then dividing it by the square root of the sample size, it is a statement of sample variability that also considers the size of the sample.

Standard deviation is the measure of the variation among a set of values. A low standard deviation indicates that the values tend to be close to the set's mean. A high standard deviation indicates that the values are spread out over a broader range (i.e., higher variability). The higher the spread of this variability, the higher the risk of operational failure.

For example, ambulance response times are proven to be an accurate predictor of patient survival as a measurable health-related outcome. The activity, "Transport affected patients from the scene to the hospital," is also measurable in binomial terms of outcome (e.g., the percentage with yes/no attributes). The same activity (i.e., process) is also measurable in performance as continuous data (e.g., number of patients transported, time-cycle, number of human resource-hours, cost, and materials). This activity is also a key indicator for medical response to disasters. A high degree of variability in ambulance response times during normal operations can be an objective predictor of response time variability during a disaster. Along with the proper mathematical **modeling**, disaster exercises offer a valuable opportunity to perform multiple trials of the same tests under controlled circumstances where performance and outcomes may be measured, analyzed, and predicted for emergency operations.

22.7.3 Six Sigma™

Six Sigma™ is derived from the bell curve used in statistics where one sigma (σ) represents one standard deviation away from the mean [99]. The defect rate is extremely low when the process exhibits six sigmas, (i.e., $\pm 3\sigma$). In other words, using six standard deviations, we can treat the information as having a 99.7 percent certainty. Put simply, we may assume with a 99.7 percent level of confidence that this value is correct.

The process control chart is typically constructed to represent the upper control limit as plus three standard deviations ($+3\sigma$) and the lower control limit as minus three standard deviations (-3σ). These upper and lower limits form the boundaries for what is an acceptable and unacceptable degree of variance. Events (i.e., tests of the EOP activity) that fall outside of the upper or lower control limits represent processes that are out of control and therefore warrant corrective action. These calculations may be performed for continuous data (e.g., X-bar and R-bar calculations measuring variability in the mean number and range of defects) and binomial attribute data (e.g., P-bar calculations measuring the proportion of defects) and counting data (C-bar measuring the number of defects per process).

These performance values are easily presentable in the form of dashboards – graphical displays of data using scales and graphics that audiences (e.g., EOP stakeholders and emergency managers) readily understand.

22.8 Process Improvement and Control

As initially introduced in Section 1.8, multiple, well-validated approaches for process improvement, including Kaizen™, Lean™, and Six Sigma™, have been developed following Deming's ground-breaking work involving TQM™ and the PDCA cycle. Chapter 23 focuses on improving and maintaining plan quality by using the Six Sigma™ DMAIC approach as a guide for process improvement and a hierarchy of controls for maintaining process control [99] (see Figure 22.1).

22.9 Case Study: Testing the Pyronesia Public Health EOP

In this case study, EOP stakeholders of Pyronesia have recently completed a National Exercise, which is held every year at Koshiba Field, the national airport. After the exercise, the planners immediately hosted a **hotwash**-style after-action review among its participants. This event typically involves the sharing of first impressions and anecdotal information regarding performance during the exercise. During this public hotwash session, the group discussed the EOP activity related to the transportation of injured patients to the hospital via ambulance. One exercise participant felt that the ambulances "ran too slowly." Another participant said that from their experience, the ambulance response was "adequate." Then, one of the volunteer patients spoke up and said that his trip was "delayed by over ten minutes" while awaiting ambulance arrival. The hotwash facilitator then asked the entire group for their impression, and it was the group's consensus that the ambulances were "a problem."

During this same exercise, the Pyronesia health ministry also sought to test their newly developed public health EOP. They had monitored the data being generated from the exercise as all the responsible parties tested their performance of the same process (i.e., transportation of patients from Koshiba Field to Dever National Hospital). They intended to perform an annual evaluation to assess variability in performance. This annual evaluation was intended to guide process improvement and reduce uncertainty related to implementing the EOP. In other words, this evaluation was also intended to evaluate the return on government investments that had been made over the past year in developing the capability and capacity (i.e., preparing) for patient transport following a **mass casualty incident** (MCI). The goal is to represent this value in terms of a metric that would justify its application (e.g., the cost-effectiveness of preparedness).

The related strategic goal is stated in the Pyronesia public health EOP as follows: "People have equal access to effective, safe and quality health services." There are several associated operational objectives. In this case, stakeholders are interested in testing their ability to treat injured disaster victims. One related operational objective is as follows: "People have access to effective injury care during disasters to prevent avoidable morbidity, mortality, and disability." And the associated activity (e.g., process) being analyzed is written in the EOP as follows, "Transport injured patients from the incident site to the hospital for care." This activity typically involves patients being rescued, triaged, stabilized, and staged for transport to the hospital by ambulance. This activity occurs during the "golden hour," that time immediately following an injury when the acuity of care becomes critically crucial for preventing morbidity, mortality, and disability. The EOP has recognized the National Service for Aid in Medical Urgencies (SAMU) as the agency with primary responsibility for delivering mass casualty care in the prehospital setting. SAMU routinely works with the National Hospital System to coordinate this transfer of patients year-round. The EOP assigns secondary responsibility for completing this activity to the Pyronesia Red Cross that actively maintains a small cadre of certified volunteers to perform first aid and basic triage. Table 22.2 provides a list of indicators, measures, and target standards of performance for this activity developed by the stakeholders for this activity.

Stakeholders began their analysis of the patient transport process with a Pareto analysis to identify the most prevalent types of defects. This analysis began by classifying each of the defects into categories that could then be tallied.

Table 22.2. Target standards, measures, and indicators of process performance for the EOP activity, "Transport injured patients from the incident site to the hospital for care"

Key performance indicator	Performance measure	Target standard
Timeliness	Transport time: Elapsed time (in minutes) between patient departure from the incident scene and arrival at the hospital	60 minutes/patient
	Cycle time: Elapsed time (in minutes) for round trip of ambulance (including patient transport to hospital and return to the scene)	150 minutes/patient
Financing	Reimbursement rate for SAMU during declared disasters	€100/patient
Completeness	Proportion of all activities assigned that were completed	100% of all activities
Efficiency	Level of resources used per activity	1 SAMU driver 1 SAMU medical technician 1 ambulance 1 trauma kit with supplies for one patient
Effectiveness	Proportion of trials with 100% on-time accomplishment	95% of trials are 100% accomplished
	Patient survival rates	80% of patients transported survive their injury
Cost effectiveness	Cost of survival per patient	€125/survival
Quality	The degree of self-reported satisfaction among stakeholders and patients	80% of respondents score quality as >3 on a 5-point Likert scale

Using transport data collected during the standardized national exercise held at the national airport, stakeholders identified thirteen different variations (i.e., performance defects) that occurred during the drills. The defects were classified as follows:

- Defect M_1 – Miscommunication between incident scene ICS and SAMU resulted in no trip.
- Defect M_2 – Miscommunication between hospital and SAMU resulted in no trip.
- Defect T_1 – Transport time (scene to the hospital).
- Defect T_2 – Late arrival of SAMU to scene.
- Defect T_3 – Long scene-hospital roundtrip cycle time.
- Defect C – Activity not completed.
- Defect E_1 – Many resources used.
- Defect E_2 – Trials that were late and not completed.
- Defect E_3 – Trials where the patient did not survive.
- Defect Q_1 – Trials with low stakeholder satisfaction scores.

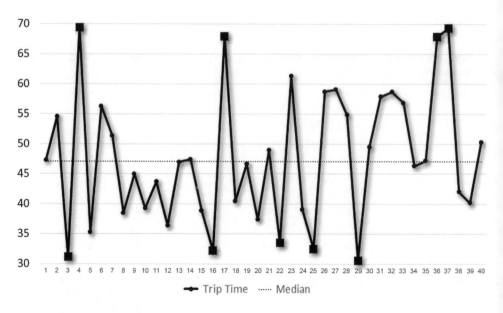

Figure 22.4 Run chart for patient transport time activity, T_1

- Defect Q_2 – Trials with low patient satisfaction scores.
- Defect F_1 – Not reimbursed due to lack of documentation.
- Defect F_2 – Not reimbursed due to non-payment.

These results are presented in Figure 22.3, illustrating the **Pareto principle** (that approximately 80 percent of costs are caused by 20 percent of defects).

According to this analysis, a minority of defects (the three related to miscommunication and scene arrival times) represent 80 percent of the low-quality cost. Pyronesia, therefore, focused its efforts on improving these three defects.

The next step was to create a process run chart that plotted the current data for each of these defects to provide a "quick and dirty" answer to whether the process is in control. In this example, stakeholders have selected defect T_1, long transport time (in minutes) from the national exercise scene at the airport to the hospital. The run chart presents the data for individual ambulance runs compared to the median value for the entire group. Figure 22.4 depicts the data used for this analysis.

Considering this run chart, stakeholders identified nine instances where the ambulance run appeared to be more variable (noted by black squares in Figure 22.4). In five instances, run times appeared much lower than the median, and in four instances, the run times were much higher. But then, what does "much higher" really mean? In other words, there was a question regarding whether this difference is significant enough to consider it a reasonable variation from the current standard (i.e., the median). To answer this question, the health ministry performed a drill – the functional test of this one activity. In this drill, fifteen ambulances were used to transport simulated patients from the Koshiba Field to nearby Dever National Hospital. Each of these ambulances completed three observed runs for which transport times were documented.

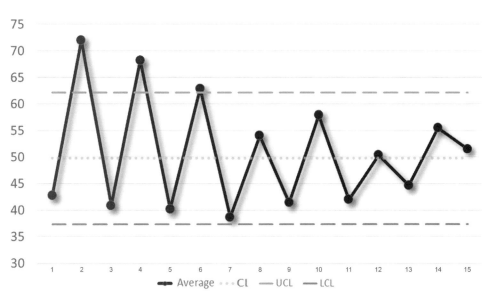

Figure 22.5 Mean patient transport times presented within upper and lower control limits of ±3 standard deviations

After completion of the drill, the health ministry created a process control chart for this EOP activity. The mean trip times for the three observed runs were calculated for each of the fifteen ambulances sampled. Two control charts were created. One chart, the X-bar (Figure 22.5), identified the centerline as the mean of the sample mean, and another chart, the R-bar (Figure 22.6), identified the centerline as the mean of the range of samples. Besides the centerline, upper, and lower (99.7 percent) confidence levels were calculated for the data. These levels were represented as dotted lines that form the upper and lower limits of the graphs (see Figures 22.5 and 22.6).

Considering this X-bar control chart in Figure 22.5, it appears that the variability in mean transport time decreased over time as each of the fifteen trips were performed. This pattern is consistent with a trend of diminishing uncertainty and the increasing likelihood of a successful outcome. According to these findings, there does not appear to be a "problem" with the ambulance that would require further remediation.

Considering the R-bar control chart in Figure 22.6, it appears that the variability in the range of transport times also decreased over time from trial #1 to trial #15. Like that for the mean times, this pattern is consistent with a diminishing uncertainty that often comes with learning and practice. These fifteen trials were performed by fifteen different EMS ambulances being managed by one transportation officer. Thus, the role of practice and learning on this transportation officer's performance may, therefore, warrant additional study. While these data explain the anecdotal experiences from the hotwash discussion, there does not appear to be a "problem" with the ambulance that would require further remediation.

In this case study, the process control analysis involved variables on a continuous scale (time). Sample size requirements are therefore smaller than for proportion data. Generally, an allowable sample size (n) is between four and ten, with twenty samples being included in the calculation. When using proportional (binomial – yes/no) data, at least twenty samples of forty items each are required to calculate P-bar, the average proportion that is defective.

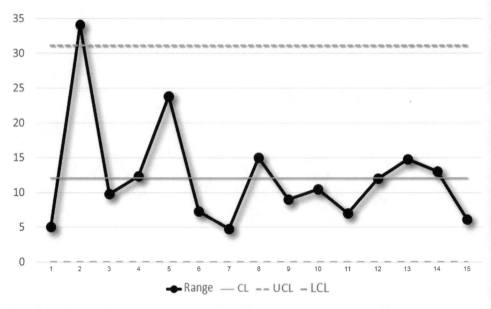

Figure 22.6 Range of patient transport times presented within upper and lower control limits of ±3 standard deviations

Finally, in the case of counting data (data measured per unit), at least twenty samples of forty items each are required to calculate C-bar, the number of defects per unit.

In each of these examples, decisions regarding changes in the EOP intended for process improvement were based upon evidence that can be calculated when considering specific, measurable, attainable, realistic, and time-based activities (see Doran's SMART objectives in Section 8.9). By using these methods, stakeholders may define, execute, and measure the effectiveness of the EOP using empirical methods that are reliably reproducible and statistically valid.

Finally, this case study measured an activity related to healthcare. But it could have just as easily been designed to test a public health activity from the EOP, such as vector surveillance. The time cycles needed to deploy and collect vector traps could be used to measure activity efficiency. Alternately, the amount of a daily water ration effectively delivered could just as easily be the object of measure for attribute data related to emergency operations. In each case, the ADEPT™ system allows for an integration of planning, execution, and control of emergency operations.

22.10 Questions for Discussion

1. Compare and contrast the value of using statistical control data for EOP decision-making with anecdotes originating from traditional "hotwash-style" after-action studies.

2. Some jurisdictions routinely integrate disaster-related measures into everyday documentation, thereby testing many of the activities of the EOP regularly. Describe how the process of disaster-related triage performed by ambulances and hospitals could be instituted, monitored, and evaluated for applicability during the disaster.

Chapter

Plan Improvement

23.1 Learning Objectives

Upon completion of the chapter, the reader can:

Define the following terms and phrases:
- Control theory
- Cost-benefit analysis
- Hierarchy of process control
- Project management triangle.

23.2 The ADEPT™ Approach to Plan Improvement

This chapter focuses on process improvement and process control. As initially introduced in Section 1.8, there are multiple, well-validated approaches available for process improvement (e.g., TQM™, Kaizen™, Lean™, and Six Sigma™). The ADEPT™ system utilizes the Six Sigma DMAIC approach (defining, measuring, analyzing, improving, and correcting) to guide process improvement and a hierarchy of controls for ensuring process control [99] (see Figure 22.1).

22.3 Process Improvement

Figure 23.1 depicts the five steps of the Six Sigma DMAIC cycle that are used to manage a process.

This model includes defining, measuring, analyzing, improving, and correcting EOP activities to ensure that events conform to the intended emergency operations plan (EOP) outcomes (i.e., operational objectives and strategic goals).

Figure 23.1 thus depicts the five steps for improving the reliability and validity of a process. The reliability of an EOP is improved by improving its reproducibility. Reproducibility is improved by using a standard model for defining the process. The SOARR™ format offers a standardized, reproducible model for defining EOP activities (i.e., processes). The validity of an EOP is improved by improving the ability to accomplish intended goals and objectives (i.e., outcomes).

The specific steps to process improvement are dependent upon the process metric being used (e.g., resources, time, scope, quality, and productivity). Once the performance indicators and metrics have been evaluated during the process analysis, decisions

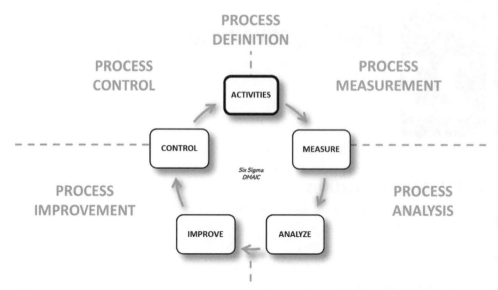

Figure 23.1 The Six Sigma DMAIC cycle as applied to process management [98]

may be made regarding corrective actions that reduce variability among those EOP activities found to be out of control.

23.4 The Project Management Triangle

The process measures of time, resources (e.g., cost), and scope have been described as interdependent upon each other in terms of quality. This **project management triangle** has been used to describe how making changes in one constraint can either affect the quality or result in a corresponding accommodation by another process measure. The familiar saying is, "Time, cost and scope – choose two!" For example, an activity can be completed in less time by increasing resources or cutting scope. Similarly, an increasing scope may require equivalent increases in resources and time. Cutting resources without adjusting time or scope will lead to lower quality. Since this balance involves a value judgment, it is best performed by consensus among EOP stakeholders responsible for its execution.

This judgment is best accomplished through O2C3-based decision-making that was also applied to writing the activity in the first place. Those parties identified in the EOP as having primary and secondary responsibility for completing the activity should also be involved in this subsequent process for improvement. These responsible parties named in the EOP are reconvened to create an objective-based plan for process improvement. This plan is known as the preparedness plan for response (PPR). The PPR intends to improve these defective processes in such a way as to reduce variability in the performance and intended outcomes of emergency response operations. Just like the EOP, the PPR is written in SOARR™ format using an O2C3 approach (see Figure 13.1).

23.5 Process Control

Control systems engineering uses **control theory** to design operational systems (like emergency operations). The practice characteristically monitors the output performance of the process being controlled. These measurements are then used as a feedback loop to guide corrective actions to achieve the desired performance.

Put simply, process control is the system of checks and balances that managers use to reduce variability so that they can ensure reliability and validity for their work. Emergency managers use process control to reduce variability and uncertainty during the implementation of the EOP. In this manner, they can ensure that activities and their resultant outcomes conform to the EOP.

Examples of different process control techniques include adaptive, intelligent, and hierarchical control. A hierarchical control system is a type of control system arranged in a hierarchical tree. This hierarchical tree employs the controls as an algorithm arranged in rank order.

This hierarchy of controls offers a layered approach for controlling the process at various levels. Process control is ranked with the highest priority given to the most effective control and lowest priority given to the least effective one. This hierarchy intends to establish preventive control over performance variability and defects ("prevention through design") [100].

Figure 23.2 depicts a hierarchy of controls as applied to process improvement.

In the case of emergency response operations, managers may apply these five levels of process control to reduce the variability among EOP activities that would otherwise result in a negative performance or outcome. Once defects in performance or outcome have been identified during the process analysis and corrected during process improvement, the preventive control principle is then applied through actions that control future variability and uncertainty.

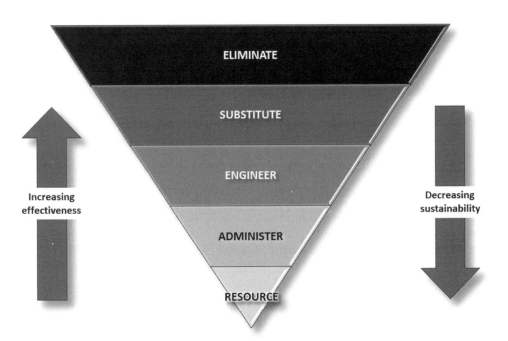

Figure 23.2 The hierarchy of process control

23.6 The Hierarchy of Process Control

The priority of hierarchical process control is to eliminate the defective process. In the case of emergency operations, stakeholders would simply delete the activity from the EOP. The corresponding objective would either be accomplished using a different tactic or eliminated. This step is critical because it is based upon recognizing that some activities are simply not achievable or reproducible *to the degree upon which it may be reliable.*

When it is not possible to eliminate the activity, stakeholders may instead substitute another activity in its place that accomplishes the same operational objective. Whenever substitution is not a viable alternative, stakeholders may then "engineer" or change the design of (i.e., re-write) the same activity to allow for less variability and uncertainty. This redesign involves a targeted reconvening of affected EOP stakeholders to redesign the activity.

In the cases where activities may not be amenable to redesign, stakeholders may choose to change how the activity is administered (e.g., managed by the ICS). Readministered activities may involve the coordination with external resources that augment or replace stakeholder capacity (e.g., mutual aid agreements, memorandums of understanding) or more intensive coordination of internal resources (e.g., strike teams and task forces).

Finally, when administrative controls are not adequate, stakeholders may choose to change how the activity is resourced (e.g., by changing staffing, funding, time, or logistical support). By adding additional resources, the stakeholders must balance effectiveness with efficiency. They must be mindful of the cost of resourcing an EOP activity versus its expected benefit. In other words, administrative controls are selected based on the expected cost-effectiveness of the intervention that they accomplish (i.e., cost/objective). Resource-based controls often sustain the highest recurring costs and require the most ongoing maintenance. They are, therefore, the most difficult to sustain over time. Anyone working in disaster logistics and inventory management can readily attest to this unfortunate fact that often serves as the bane of their existence.

23.7 Cost-Benefit Analysis

As a general rule for cost-effectiveness, the best choices are those that eliminate the activity (and its associated uncertainty) altogether and therefore acquire no recurring costs (or ongoing risk of failure) associated with their implementation. The least effective of these controls require a recurring expenditure of resources to maintain preventive control over adverse performance or outcomes. The more resource-intensive controls are the least cost-effective. They are more difficult to sustain because they do not establish "prevention through design" as a default. Adding additional resources to improve a defective activity's performance is therefore considered an option of last resort for process control. Unfortunately, this may be the first inclination of some stakeholders (e.g., "to throw more money/resources at the problem") during a crisis. A better approach is to apply the scientific method to compare the relative cost and benefit of these interventions. The hierarchy of process control offers one approach for selecting the most cost-effective process controls for emergency operations.

23.8 Case Study: Improving Medical Surge Capacity in Pyronesia

As part of its ongoing commitment to national emergency preparedness, the Pyronesia health ministry regularly hosts a national public health and medical exercise, each year focusing on a different capability in the public health EOP. This year the focus is on the EOP core capability of medical surge as related to mass casualty incidents (MCIs) (see Table 4.3).

The US Centers for Disease Control and Prevention (CDC) describes the public health capability of medical surge as "the ability to provide adequate medical evaluation and care during events that exceed the limits of the normal medical infrastructure of an affected community" [101].

In follow-up to testing the national EOP during the national airport exercise, the health ministry performed a process analysis for the EOP objective, "The surge capacity for transportation of injured patients is increased by 30% above the limits of normal SAMU operations." This objective is accomplished by several activities, one of which is already in the EOP, "Transport injured patients using the entire fleet of (60) SAMU ambulances."

This activity was tested by way of a real event that involved simultaneous notification and activation of all SAMU ambulances for a rail accident at Martha's Garden, the nation's largest tourist destination. There were over 300 casualties estimated on the initial count. Ambulance arrival and dispatch times to and from Martha's Garden were documented, as were the ambulance arrival and departure times from the Dever National Hospital located near the airport on the opposite side of the country (two hours by ground). The event resulted in the transportation of twenty patients during the first two hours, then forty patients during the third hour, after which the rate of patient transport occurred at only ten patients per hour. At the end of the twelve hour-long event, only 150 patients had been transported. This number represented approximately half of the average number of ambulance runs on a typical (nondisaster) day! This disaster uncovered an operational bottleneck that prevented the successful accomplishment of the intended outcome (i.e., medical surge capacity). This bottleneck occurred during the staging of patients at the incident site in preparation for transport.

Stakeholders have now reconvened to improve this activity (i.e., process) with the context of a set of controls that reduce the likelihood of this same defect (e.g., a drop in SAMU patient capacity) occurring in the future.

Stakeholders utilized process management first to define a new process (i.e., draft a new EOP activity), create a plan for its improvement (i.e., draft a new PPR activity), and then implement measures that control future outcomes and include "prevention by design."

Stakeholders begin their deliberation by brainstorming for ways to improve the process. They consider the first level in the hierarchy of controls, elimination of the activity. Since the level of process performance is currently unacceptable, stakeholders ask themselves, "Is it possible to delete the activity altogether without affecting the intended outcome?" (e.g., that "The surge capacity for transportation of injured patients is increased by 30 percent above the limits of normal SAMU operations"). The answer is no. The national risk assessment has identified multiple hazards (including rail accidents) that could result in up to 300 casualties.

In that case, the next choice is for stakeholders to consider whether other activities may be substituted for (or added to) the EOP activity, "Transport injured patients using the entire fleet of (60) SAMU ambulances." Several stakeholders propose potential substitutions that may also add other means of patient transport (e.g., air, rail, as well as using non-ambulance private vehicles). Others propose the utilization of closer hospitals for less severe patients who do not require Dever National Hospital's advanced care. Other stakeholders noted that the patient staging and loading systems could be better engineered at the incident scene for more efficient ambulance traffic (e.g., barriers that better control vehicle ingress and egress into future MCI scenes). The group also identified a system for organizing the flow of vehicles away from the site that would match the level of patient acuity to the appropriate hospital according to both bed availability and patient severity. This system is currently used at one hospital and could be extended to others. And finally, some proposed that the private vehicles of over 400 SAMU employees could be resourced with a basic life support kit (i.e., enough materials for treatment of trauma patient). These resources could then be used to augment the current shift of ambulance workers already called to the site.

These ideas were documented as they were proposed during the brainstorming session. Each process was defined as an activity that could offer a viable hypothesis to be tested (see Figure 1.2). These tests are used to identify the most valid, reliable, and cost-effective courses of action from among these proposed options.

23.9 Questions for Discussion

Describe an experiment (i.e., exercise) that would test the above-proposed options for process control, as related to the Pyronesia national public health and medical exercise:

- elimination,
- substitution,
- substitution,
- engineering,
- administration, and
- resourcing.

Chapter

Planning Pitfalls

24.1 Learning Objectives

Upon completion of the chapter, the reader can:

1. Define the following terms and phrases:
   - 6W1H approach
   - Bloom's taxonomy
   - Cognitive reframing
   - Community readiness
   - Frame of reference
   - Governance.
2. List the upper three levels for each of the following domains from Bloom's taxonomy of learning: psychomotor, cognitive, and affective.
3. Recognize common planning pitfalls related to governance, methodology, stakeholdership, and inclusion.
4. Describe the importance of matching an intervention to a community's level of readiness.
5. Compare the SOARR™ format to the 6W1H approach to information gathering.
6. Describe how cognitive reframing can be used to redirect negative perceptions related to the EOP stakeholder's frame of reference.

24.2 Planning Is Learning

Like any process, the act of planning is not without its pitfalls. As mentioned in Chapter 5, the process itself is complex and labor-intensive. After studying the process of disaster planning involving the development of literally hundreds of plans, a handful of issues appear to arise during disaster planning regardless of language, nationality, sector, or type of plan.

Stakeholders should be aware of these common challenges that often occur in association with emergency operations planning. It can help identify potential sources of contention, obstruction, or inattention that are most likely to affect the planning process's performance and outcome.

It is essential to recognize that planning itself is a learning experience. As introduced in Figure 21.1, insights gained from the interpretation of information leads to new knowledge – a new actionable "rule" that can then, in turn, be applied to other information. A positive feedback loop for learning also exists between information and knowledge. Thus,

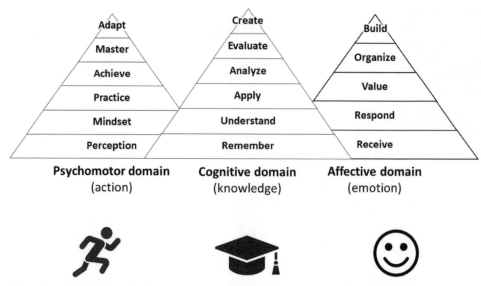

Figure 24.1 Bloom's revised taxonomy as applied to cognitive, affective, and psychomotor learning

the better we learn, the better we plan (which results in better learning). As stakeholders gather and process data and information, they gain additional knowledge and understanding to predict the future with some reasonable degree of certainty. This act involves more than merely the creation of a shared document. Planning thus involves learning. And not merely learning, but effective planning requires the highest learning levels across three separate domains (e.g., cognitive, affective, and psychomotor). Figure 24.1 depicts **Bloom's taxonomy**, a hierarchical model that describes the various learning levels that occur across these three domains of human endeavor.

In effect, emergency operations plan (EOP) stakeholders are expected to operate at the highest three levels of learning (noted in grey at the top of each pyramid in Figure 24.1) as they:

- achieve, master, and adapt the skills needed to,
- value collaboration, organize themselves, and build consensus for,
- analysis, evaluation, and creation of an effective plan.

Therefore, planning should be treated as a comprehensive learning process where most stakeholders begin at the very bottom of these three pyramids and then, during the planning process, learn how to plan together as a group. Stakeholders must be allowed to remember, understand, and apply their knowledge before being expected to analyze, evaluate, and create. They must first understand their operating environment and the mindset for planning before they can practice, then become proficient and then master the planning process. Finally, stakeholders must also learn stakeholdership itself – the level of personal and emotional commitment that comes through being emotionally receptive in a way that helps to solidify involvement and build value.

Community readiness is a model for change that integrates a community's culture, resources, and readiness level to more effectively address an issue [102]. Matching an intervention to a community's level of readiness is essential for success. Interventions must be challenging enough to move a community forward in its level of readiness without being overwhelming.

Readiness allows stakeholders to define issues and strategies in their contexts and build cooperation among systems and individuals. Efforts must, therefore, be given to developing an educational approach to the planning process. The outcome of planning is a form of "group intelligence" that EOP stakeholders first share, then learn, and then apply to predict the future.

This chapter discusses the most common pitfalls associated with emergency operations planning. These challenges may be categorized into four main groups related to governance, methodology, stakeholdership, and inclusion. A framework is also offered for considering potential solutions to these pitfalls. Using this framework, planners are prompted to answer a series of simple questions that help identify and reframe the discussion.

24.3 Planning Pitfalls Related to Governance

Planning pitfalls related to governance include a mandate, project staffing, cross-sectoral collaboration, program management, and leadership. As discussed in Chapter 15, a mandate is an essential prerequisite for effective emergency operation planning. Planners require an apparent authority along with a clear responsibility. The support of the chief executive should be explicitly stated and demonstrated. This high-level of support communicates the strategic importance of the mission and the vision for its application. An official mandate also attracts the appropriate people to the planning process. As stated in Chapter 10, it is essential to have the "right people in the room" when writing a plan.

An executive order is beneficial when seeking to convene leaders from across the entire institution. It is often deemed nearly impossible to convene a large group of managers from across an institution or governmental agency for the sake of planning. Managers are, by nature, preoccupied with current operations. However, it is, in fact, relatively straightforward when the will and mandate exist.

During one project that I led at CDC, we convened nearly 100 leaders across the CDC, including the directors of centers, laboratories, divisions, and branches, to write a plan for radiation emergencies. This level of support occurred after we all received a direct letter from the CDC Director. In another project in Mauritius, I led a hospital planning project that convened the administrators and leadership from all fourteen regional hospitals in the country. In a different project in another (un-named) country, the provincial chief executive began their speech at the opening ceremony as follows, "Today, we will plan. You will plan, or you will be punished." My translator responded to my look of amazement only with a smile and an affirmative nod. The degree of commitment can be remarkable when the importance of the mandate is made clear!

Good **governance** also occurs through consistent staffing of the planning program on an ongoing basis. Good governance allows for planning to occur across sectors, across administrations, and across political parties. Good governance is also required for program sustainability. Preparedness programs depend upon consistent governance over time. Planning must be instituted as part of a comprehensive preparedness program and not merely a project. Finally, good governance requires accountable leadership. In addition to establishing a mandate, leaders are also responsible for the successful implementation of the EOP. However, many leaders do not like plans because they serve to document workers' roles and responsibilities and the measures of performance for the leaders themselves. The common complaint about performance management, "You can't measure what I do," is all too often uttered by managers that in effect, "do little" [11].

Many of us have had a boss afflicted by the so-called shiny object syndrome. It has been described as a continual state of distraction among managers. It often comes at the expense of what is already planned or underway. It has been posited as rooted in the childhood phenomenon of always wanting a new toy or as a means for the ambitious manager to constantly maneuver themselves to present the highest visibility to their boss, the chief executive. This tactic involves a routine of always "going" where their boss is "looking" rather than creating measurable accomplishments that attract the boss' attention.

I once worked for a manager that preferred to work nearly exclusively in "shiny object" tasks – decided ad hoc and assigned on a first-come, first-served basis. Unfortunately, by the time the first set of tasks were reported back to the manager, they were rarely ever met with the same level of enthusiasm with which they were delegated. And by the time for a second update, the manager had usually lost all interest in the task entirely (or was on business travel). Besides the fact that the activities rarely ever ended in some measurable outcome, the process used to get there was also toxic to most stakeholders involved (perhaps excluding the manager).

Not surprisingly, during the same time, the same manager received repeated urgings from their own supervisor to develop a strategic plan for the office to help them organize the group better. After finally acquiescing, the office developed an impressive annual work plan engaging the entire staff and leadership's input. Once created, the shiny object manager shared it with their supervisor for positive (i.e., shiny) feedback. However, the plan was never instituted in the office. And within three years, half the staff and the manager were gone. Sound familiar? The point is that planning is one of the five fundamental roles of management.

Managers that cannot plan, cannot manage.

24.4 Planning Pitfalls Related to the Methodology

There are several pitfalls associated with the methodology used for planning. Most of these challenges stem from the temptation to bypass the scientific method and implement hypotheses rather than evidence (see Figure 1.1). While it may appear expedient in the short-term, this missed step can have enormous long-term implications concerning the plan's performance and outcome. Pressed by resource constraints, planners may fail to use exercises as experiments that create actionable intelligence. They may be tempted to replace experiential evidence documented through quantitative testing of the EOP with the more expedient anecdote and opinions voiced through after-action reviews. They may view the time spent on process improvement as a low priority for program *maintenance* compared to an investment opportunity for program *growth*. Finally, there is the problem that "we don't have the data because we don't collect the data." This paucity makes it easy to throw up one's hands and say that all processes associated with public health and medical emergency operations are somehow immeasurable or too complicated. However, similar advances routinely occur within these disciplines when applied to issues that are not related to disasters.

24.5 Planning Pitfalls Related to Stakeholdership

The third group of planning pitfalls, lack of stakeholdership, is also related to the other categories of challenges. Stakeholdership is a fundamental requirement of effective planning and is consistent with the current level of commitment required by governance. However, stakeholdership extends beyond compliance into empowerment. With ownership and accountability come a sense of risk- sharing, resource-sharing, and sharing the resultant credit for accomplishments. This sense of ownership allows stakeholders to develop a mutual trust committed to a "partnership of equals" and producing outcomes of value to the entire community (not just the "official" organizations) [27, 43]. The use of consensus-based decision-making during the planning process allows for equitable partnerships during this process – an essential element of community satisfaction and risk perception.

24.6 Planning Pitfalls Related to Inclusion

It is within this context of stakeholdership that the importance of inclusion is brought to bear. Some are tempted to classify all emergency plans as confidential in the age of information security and fusion centers. They oddly posit that somehow a potential adversary would have to know more about the local earthquake or tornado plan to make an effective attack on national security. There may also be the temptation to include only public assets in the plan, thereby ignoring the source of the majority of community capacity – that of the private sector. Plans that focus inordinately on official versus unofficial agencies often tend to centralize and propagate "official" power rather than empowering the community to be an equal partner in the solution. According to a narrow perspective, even within official channels, so-called silos of excellence too often typify the application of emergency management. Many times, managers are tempted to bypass community engagement while justifying their actions as expedient. While appearing more straightforward, this same approach may, at the same time, forestall any possibility of a successful outcome. Finally, according to the Sphere Project humanitarian standards, it is essential for the people being served by an emergency response to have a voice in its design and implementation [103]. For this reason, the community should be involved in every step of disaster planning, not merely during the exercise. There is remarkable value in identifying individuals and groups within the community that represent both the formal and informal leadership – society's network and fabric. These faith-based organizations, nongovernmental charities, private companies, and individual families form the real value, the "silver lining" of arduous planning – the network that is created. For this reason, those who write the plan should also include those who are served by the plan. And those who execute the plan should also be representative of the community's norms, culture, and diversity.

24.7 Avoiding the Pitfalls

24.7.1 Stay the Course

This book describes a system for planning that is deliberately designed to avoid many of these most common pitfalls. However, no system is *useful* if it is not *used*. And it is tempting for some participants to change the planning process rather than change their frames of reference – even though these changes may be self-defeating. Over the past two decades, I have worked with many individuals who, upon attending their first few hours of a planning workshop, seek to redesign the entire process to align with their professional perspective, mental constructs (or personal ambition).

It may also be tempting to substitute a different nomenclature for explaining the process of planning. This book is full of definitions that planners must first recognize, understand, and then apply – many times during their first encounter. It may appear more comfortable to fall back upon old habits and outdated definitions. As words are interpreted differently by different individuals, they may wish to "rename" some of the components or "reframe" some of the definitions. This act offers a slippery slope toward a nonstandardized, immeasurable, and nonreproducible plan.

Thus, the advice for avoiding these pitfalls is simple, "Use the system." And to use the system, one must first learn it. Take the time to understand the definitions, the scientific models, the management approaches, and the analyses that go into administering an efficient and effective plan. Invest the time now for a return that grows exponentially later. More time spent learning pays long-term dividends in terms of your improved efficiency, effectiveness, and satisfaction.

24.7.2 Cognitive Reframing

One of the challenges involved in implementing a planning process that is highly inclusive and diverse in its representation is related to managing the pitfalls that are commonly associated with group learning and decision-making. This "bringing together of brains" involves developing consensus through a process of learning and planning. People are "learning how to learn together – then learning how to plan together," so to speak.

This level of collaboration draws upon multiple frames of reference from each of the participants. Bolman and Deal identified four frames of reference from which organizations may be viewed [104]. The *structural frame* involves defined roles, specific responsibilities, and formal roles of constituents within the organization. The *human resource frame* is more deeply rooted in the affective domain of learning, involving an individual's feelings and emotions. The *political frame* relates to the common thread of conflict inherent to any negotiation process among different groups (as members of an organization advance their agendas). Finally, organizations also rely upon a *symbolic frame* of reference to characterize the collection of events, traditions, and histories that identify and distinguish one group from another.

It may be helpful for planners to be on the watch for signs of dysfunctional frames of reference among the stakeholders as planning unfolds. The structural frame is often the least practical approach for reaching a mutual understanding and a common perspective of an issue. Stakeholders may understand the roles and responsibilities of a plan (i.e., structural frame of reference) without recognizing negative biases or defective reasoning related to issues that are also emotional, political, or symbolic of a deeper meaning. These biases add a higher degree of uncertainty regarding the successful performance and outcome of the plan.

For this reason, it may be helpful for planners to utilize **cognitive reframing**, a discussion intended to help stakeholders alter their perceptions of a negative, distorted of self-defeating belief to change behaviors and improve planning outcomes. "Reframing is a technique used by psychologists in cognitive behavioral therapy to change the focus of a situation or problem and examine it from a different perspective. It involves looking at the reciprocal side of an issue or analyzing a situation from a broader sense" [105, p. 365].

Table 24.1. A comparison of the SOARR™ and the 6W1H formats for information gathering

Strategic goal (S)	Operational objective (O)	Activity (A)	Responsible party (R)	Resource (R)
Why?	What?	How? Where? When?	Who?	With what?

Frames of reference may also help facilitators diagnose what may appear to be negative or self-defeating behaviors during the group planning sessions. All plan stakeholders should be aware of these four frames of reference and avoid related pitfalls during the planning session.

Structural frames represent a comfortable starting point for addressing the deeper emotional, political, or symbolic issues that are less likely to be resolved in a (very) public forum. In some cases, merely reframing (and simplifying) the structural language used to describe the planning process can be helpful (particularly when planning is performed in multiple languages). Table 24.1 reveals the association between the ADEPT SOARR™ plan format and the **6W1H** model for information gathering and problem-solving.

If stakeholders reach a significant impasse (or delay in decision-making) regarding a critical requirement of the EOP, the facilitator may wish to reframe the goal, objective, activity, personnel, or resource in simpler terms. Here, the intent is not to force consensus but rather to open a new discussion line that reframes the issue from a different procedural, emotional, political, or symbolic perspective. The strategy is to first broaden the discussion before later converging again toward a final decision. During this time, the facilitator should be somewhat lenient with group members who need to discuss emotions, politics, or symbolism during these sessions. In some cases, it is one or more of these nonstructural frames of reference that are causing the pitfall. Stakeholders must feel that their concerns (including unspoken beliefs and attitudes) are addressed. Sometimes these concerns must be reframed within a trust and mutual respect for the emotions, politics, and symbolic memory that each stakeholder brings to the table. Managing stakeholder frames of reference also recognizes the inherently human aspect of planning and the value of this diversity of thought. The system may benefit from a network effect where more participants increase the plan's value without incurring an additional cost for participation.

24.8 Questions for Discussion

Given an example of the following objective: "All citizens wear facemasks in public," discuss the potential effect of the following three frames of reference on stakeholder ability to make decisions regarding the structural frame (e.g., stakeholder roles and responsibilities):

- the human resource (emotion),
- the political frame (conflict), and
- the symbolic frame (identity).

The Future of Disaster Planning

25

25.1 Learning Objectives

Upon completion of the chapter, the reader can:

1. Define the following terms and phrases:

   - Agent
   - Artificial intelligence
   - Automated planning
   - Cooperative multi-agent system
   - Machine learning
   - Network effect
   - Public health 3.0
   - Rational agent
   - Rationality
   - Semantic Web 3.0
   - Social Web 2.0
   - Standard model
   - Task networking.

2. Describe the interactions between a rational agent and the environment that occur in an intelligent operations system in terms of actuators, sensors, and the task environment.
3. Describe the relationships between Webs 1.0, 2.0, and 3.0.
4. Describe the role of public health officials in Public health 3.0.
5. List the challenges and opportunities related to the future of planning in terms of:

   - Assessing planning assumptions
   - Creating mission area plans
   - Checking planning assumptions
   - Creating preparedness plans
   - Testing mission area plans.

25.2 The Future of Disaster Planning Is a Network

This book was written during a time of remarkable global upheaval, directly impacted by rapidly advancing technologies. Advances in communications and transportation have influenced a trend of globalization, which, in turn, has made it possible for one single virus to rapidly circumnavigate the entire world. Concerning information and communication technology, the challenge is no longer a lack of data but rather searching for useful intelligence among an inundation of data. Concerns over data security are growing, and the role of digital misinformation has become a common topic of many conversations.

The way we conceive of software has changed radically. Cloud computing and software as a service are turning high-powered supercomputing into a utility that is widely available to the public. Many organizations routinely manage massive data sets (i.e., big data). Data analytics and operational intelligence drive innovation and redefine modern telecommunications, marketing, entertainment, science, engineering, the arts, and education.

Most notably, our access to Internet information is also changing. The creator-generated content and hierarchical culture of Web 1.0 have been replaced by a peer-to-peer culture of user-generated content, known as Web 2.0. Web 2.0 allows users to routinely interact and collaborate as part of a virtual community (i.e., stakeholders with a common goal).

This **social web 2.0** is now being augmented by a **semantic web 3.0**, where content has been tagged (i.e., made relational) so that the meaning can be recognized and processed by machines [106]. The goal of the semantic Web is to make Internet data machine-readable so that machines may exchange information more readily. Put simply, this involves "machines talking to machines" on the so-called internet of things. These networks represent the technological mimicry of the thinking, logic, and structures related to neuroscience. In effect, these networks are "bringing our brains together" as they ease and simplify our ability to communicate at an increasingly more detailed level of granularity, with an exponential growth in depth.

These interactive social and semantic models of the Web are occurring when recent stressors on public health are driving many local governments to pioneer a new **public health 3.0** model. In public health 3.0, public health officials serve as "chief health strategists," partnering across multiple sectors and leveraging data and resources to focus on improving the social determinants of health [107]. This model stresses the value of a **network effect**.

The convergence of these trends will undoubtedly result in innovative models for the study, implementation, and communication of effective public health interventions. The strength of these advances lies in their "network effects" (also known as Metcalfe's law) when the service becomes more valuable as more people use it [108].

When I first invented the ADEPT™ planning system in 2000, I laughingly claimed to have "advanced disaster planning all the way into the 1980s!" And what I meant by that is related to the fact that by 2000, many institutions and methodologies were already relying upon twenty-first-century technology. However, in the case of disaster planning, we were still typing out written plans and distributing them as document files – hundreds of pages (that no one ever took the time to read)! In 2000, the first step was to move disaster planning from "paper" to "electrons." Disaster planning joined the digital age twenty years ago by merely becoming a sortable and searchable relational database.

The next challenge is to move disaster planning from the "electron" to the "web," where Metcalfe's network effect may realize further gains. There, more people may gain value by utilizing a network of standardized plans, and, in return, the network becomes more intelligent and more valuable to everyone.

The *network* is more important than the plan!

This quote describes the value of the network effect in that it not only provides the "how-to" information typically contained in plans. It also includes a standard model and mechanism for comparing performance by the end-users of the plan (i.e., participants in the network). Each time one member of the network uses their plan, they create meaningful data that may be analyzed to benefit the entire network. Data sets are more likely to be robust and, therefore, more suitable for investigating statistically significant defects in plan performance across a large population. This chapter discusses some of the challenges and opportunities related to the future of disaster planning. It does so within the context of the five phases of the ADEPT™ planning wheel (see Figure 14.1).

25.3 The Future of Disaster Planning Is Automated

In the future, machines will write most plans, including disaster plans. For this reason, future disaster planners need to become familiar with some of the basic concepts of artificial intelligence (AI).

One of the many reasons that machines are so adept at planning (pun intended) is that computers can "think" more rationally than humans. Rationality is a foundational concept for understanding AI [108]. It refers to the tendency to select an action that is expected to maximize performance. A **rational agent** acts to achieve the best outcome, or, when there is uncertainty, the best-expected outcome [109]. Simply put, a rational agent is one that "does the right thing." The "right thing to do" is defined by the plan objective. This standard approach is also called the **standard model**.

In AI, an **agent** is specifically defined as "any system that perceives its environment through sensors and acts upon the environment through actuators" [109]. Thus, a rational agent acts upon its environment to achieve the standard model and monitors that environment through a series of measurable indicators. Figure 25.1 depicts an intelligent system's operations that interact with environments through sensors and actuators.

This system is the same system-based approach to operations as introduced initially in Figure 7.1, now with added feedback loops representing the bidirectional flow of data used to both monitor the objective and act upon it. This same system also forms the basis for process control theory. In other words, it is now possible for plans to learn from their own mistakes and make rapid improvements in near real-time that ensure preventive control of ongoing operations.

According to parameters that include the performance measure, environment, actuators, and sensors, these rational agents are built by specifying the task environment.

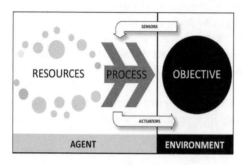

Figure 25.1 An intelligent operations system includes interactions between a rational agent and the environment

DISASTER🛡DOC

In emergency operations, the agent may be an ambulance with a performance measure of turnaround time. Sensors may include personnel, clocks, speedometers, two-way radios, telephones, accelerometers, and a global positioning system (GPS) located in each ambulance and at the emergency operations center (EOC) and field command posts, all connected by the Internet. Actuators can include personnel, two-way radios, smartphones, and the Internet. It is now possible for machines to compare field-based progress reports to the emergency operations plan (EOP) as the standard model for operations. The system may also then affect changes in the environment that result in the intended objective. These changes are accomplished by communication of actionable intelligence and operations management (i.e., planning, organizing, staffing, leading, and controlling).

25.4 Assessing Planning Assumptions

25.4.1 Challenges

Some of the current challenges related to assessing planning assumptions include (1) an absence of exposure science and (2) lack of quantitative data related to health determinants and risk factors for morbidity and mortality.

Exposure science has yet to become integrated into public health analysis associated with most disaster hazards. To date, most public health systems do not attempt to measure exposure data for the victims of most disaster hazards. (Most disaster epidemiological investigations still focus almost exclusively on demographic factors (e.g., age, gender, race, ethnicity, socio-economic status) and then lump them together under the broad (informal) case definition of "vulnerability." This myopic focus is counterproductive since it implicates social attributes as the primary cause of disaster-related health impact, rather than a reflection of colinear disaster-related exposures.

Unfortunately, advances regarding the measurement of hazardous exposures and their resultant health impacts have not kept pace with corresponding hazard analysis advancements. To date, most tools currently in use for estimation of disaster-related health impact lack statistical validity and reliability. Most historical records are incomplete or of an insufficient amount to allow for an accurate probabilistic analysis.

Health determinants and risk and protective factors remain intermixed within a relatively non-differentiated set of nomenclature that includes attribution of health effects to polysemous, nonmedical terms such as resilience and vulnerability. This lack of measurable indicators precludes any analysis that may offer a valid and reliable predictive value. This point remains of significant detriment to the accurate prediction and modeling of future health effects.

25.4.2 Opportunities

There are also significant opportunities related to the assessment of planning assumptions. These opportunities include developing standardized indices like the US National Risk Index and PreventionWeb™ country data for hazard analysis. These advances have lessened uncertainty regarding planning for the frequency and magnitude of disaster hazards worldwide. There are opportunities to standardize these measures further and increase their availability among disaster planners, especially in low resource jurisdictions. There are opportunities to apply quantitative risk analysis (now being routinely used for evaluation of chemical, biological, or radiological hazards) to a broader range of disaster hazards. There are also opportunities to integrate better dose reconstruction and other related environmental health exposure modeling efforts into risk assessments for the more common natural disaster hazards, such as floods and storms. Most public health agencies have applied only limited interventions toward injury prevention related to natural disaster hazards (other than that intended for the responders' occupational health and safety and injuries sustained during cleanup).

25.5 Creating Mission Area Plans

25.5.1 Challenges

Significant challenges also exist for creating mission area plans. These challenges include the need for (1) improved planning expertise and (2) target capability levels for mission areas of prevention, protection, and mitigation.

Most evident among these challenges is the recently recognized need to improve our expertise in planning for all mission areas. Surprisingly, when the entire planet is experiencing a pandemic disaster, there remains a paucity of guidance available for public health emergency planning (and disaster planning, in general).

As introduced in Chapter 3, most recently, the model for emergency management has been redesigned to include five mission areas that ensure preparedness for every phase (i.e., prevention, protection, mitigation, response, and recovery). This change in perspective will take some time to implement this policy as a full set of five mission area plans.

25.5.2 Opportunities

Opportunities for creating mission area plans include (1) using a systems-based approach to planning, (2) application of quality improvement principles, and (3) integration into networks that integrate **machine learning**, **automated planning**, and process control theory.

If this book has not accomplished any other objective, I hope that it will at least open the reader's eyes to the realm of opportunities that now exist for innovative planners. Using a system-based approach that integrates business administration principles, emergency management, and information technology, tomorrow's disaster planners will undoubtedly create better emergency operation plans. Of course, they will create plans and hierarchies of plans that create task networks among the stakeholders. They will design platforms that integrate multi-sectoral planning for cooperation among multiple intelligent agents and interact within a hierarchical control system. There are opportunities to apply well-established systems for process improvement, such as Deming's Total Quality Management™ and the Six Sigma model™, for process improvement. These systems will contribute quantifiable measures of success that can be derived from exercises that were otherwise based only upon hypothetical simulation and anecdote. Advances in artificial intelligence related to automated planning will allow for a more streamlined user interface and search algorithms. Finally, when machines talk to machines during the execution of emergency operations, there is less burden left to the responder for reporting quantifiable measures of efficiency and effectiveness. The use of a semantic web will allow for the automated capture of person, place, time, and process – key indicators of operational performance and applied epidemiology.

25.6 Checking Planning Assumptions

25.6.1 Challenges

Challenges related to validating planning assumptions mainly involve the lack of experience in writing five separate mission area plans that each must be associated with a preparedness plan for that mission. There is currently limited guidance for the process of a gap analysis that would identify the difference between current capacity and the level capacity that is predicted to be most likely needed for a future event.

As previously mentioned, preparedness as a crosscutting function applied to all five mission areas is a relatively new perspective. For that reason, we may also expect that public health officials have little experience in performing gap analyses that involve the capabilities and capacities associated with emergency response (let alone protection and prevention). This lack of a standardized approach also introduces another element of potential uncertainty when predicting future needs and resources.

25.6.2 Opportunities

Opportunities for checking plan assumptions include the following: (1) the standardization of target capabilities, (2) a planning network that can share and aggregate process improvement data, and (3) an improved ability for preventive control of emergency operations.

While there is little guidance available for comprehensive public health planning, there are multiple resources available to identify capabilities related to public health emergency response. These could be better standardized and communicated among public health agencies.

As mentioned in Chapter 17, due to the relative rarity of many of these events, many jurisdictions lack adequate data upon which to make evidence-based decisions. There is an opportunity to gain from the network effect if the execution of multiple jurisdictional plans were to be connected to provide reporting of aggregate data. Exercises that would usually require months to years to collect sufficient sample data could become more rapidly informed by multiple jurisdictions that perform the same activity. A comparison of this activity value to the mean value for the entire system can provide an early opportunity to detect trends that, in the past, have indicated a high probability of future defects as a result. And rather than carrying these activities out to the point of failure, machine learning would allow for each of the new values to be compared to a standard model. Trends in variance may be automatically monitored, reported, and then analyzed in real-time. Alternate choices could then be made to either eliminate the system, substitute a different activity, or search decision trees for corrective actions that will improve the outcome that better aligns with the standard model described as a process in the plan (e.g., EOP activity).

25.7 Creating Preparedness Plans

25.7.1 Challenges

There is currently limited information regarding preparedness planning that disaster planners may use to guide this critical effort. It will be necessary for planners to develop the knowledge skills and abilities (KSAs) necessary to create preparedness plans that correlate with each of these five mission areas. It will also be necessary to further develop the target capabilities and strategic goals related to those newer and lesser developed mission areas (e.g., prevention and protection).

25.7.2 Opportunities

Perhaps one of the most significant accomplishments of the past decade regarding preparedness is developing a national US policy that integrates preparedness into planning for each of the five mission areas (see Section 2.3). Up until now, most jurisdictions have created only one preparedness plan intended only for a response. Stakeholders can now develop more specific and measurable preparedness plans that apply to each of the five mission areas.

25.8 Testing Mission Area Plans

25.8.1 Challenges

Challenges related to testing mission area plans are mostly related to their lack of proven reliability and validity. Many of the means used for testing mission area plans are based upon anecdotes and tiny test samples. Few standards also involve measures of efficiency, productivity, or effectiveness. Data emanating from simulations and exercises are rarely followed and aggregated over time or according to a standard set of indicators. The result is a system that operates mainly in the absence of preventive control and process improvement over time. Put simply, we are driving the response ambulance forward to the next scene by looking in the rear-view mirror at our previous swerves and crashes.

25.8.2 Opportunities

Perhaps one of the most important messages of this book is that the testing of mission area plans represents an enormous opportunity to learn operational effectiveness from the people doing the work.

In the past, disaster planning was performed by a centralized committee comprised predominantly of institutional leadership. These upper- and middle-level managers then typically decided on the range and depth of activities that would be performed. Not surprisingly, many of these plans lacked operational detail and, as a result, were less useful to responders. Also, not surprisingly, EOPs fell out of disuse, leaving the on-scene incident managers to rely upon tactical level incident action plans to perform the real work of emergency guidance. While this decentralization of planning serves to empower incident managers to respond expeditiously, it also hampered efforts to collect aggregate data regarding these activities, which could better inform local anecdotal decision-making with national level evidence-based policies and procedures.

The ADEPT™ planning system is designed to bridge this gap between strategic policy and technical practicality. However, it is intended to do more than that. It is also intended to bridge the gap between anecdote and evidence – to apply **artificial intelligence** (AI) to help us better predict future disaster events and our related readiness to manage them.

The design of the ADEPT™ is intended to create an AI platform, a cooperative, **multi-agent** system for hierarchical **automated planning** and **task networking** that also includes a feedback loop for machine learning and process control.

The SOARR™ data schema creates a "standard model" AI structure for the EOP and, as a hierarchical data structure, it also allows for alignment with AI search trees and learning algorithms that describe the relationships between the plan's current and future inputs and outputs.

Digital platforms have now made this capability readily accessible to the masses. Stakeholders may now convene (even virtually) to assess, plan, check, prepare, and test mission area plans using the most up-to-date approaches and technology. They may now take full advantage of the cloud's enormous computing power to build libraries of data regarding the effectiveness and efficiency of plan execution related to individual EOP activities and target capabilities and objectives. These libraries may now be accessed and analyzed from all corners of the world to be applied at the national macro (EOP) and the local micro (incident action plan, IAP) level. There is no longer any excuse for misguided or uninformed leadership to claim a lack of expertise or technology regarding disaster-related interventions' success. From measurement comes certainty. From certainty comes success. And from our success comes our safety.

> It is not good enough to "do good." We must "do good" well.
> And to "do good" well, we must plan
>
> – Mark Keim

25.9 Case Study: The Partners for Information Exchange (PIE) Program

The nation of Pyronesia has embarked upon a new regional project in partnership with its bordering neighbors. The new Partners for Information Exchange (PIE) goal is to develop projects that use simple applications of artificial intelligence toward solving real-world problems related to emergency management. Pyronesia has recently been awarded a grant to investigate methods for improving its response to a long-standing source of disaster-related morbidity and mortality. The health ministry has chosen to study the National Emergency Medical System (NEMS) response to a recurrent mass casualty incident (MCI) that occurs at Malin's Cliff near the eastern border.

The Malins' Cliff area has become notorious over the years as a common source of multiple vehicle accidents. During the past decade, there have been multiple reports of MCIs, many associated with the cross-border bus traffic that weaves its way through a narrow mountainous roadway. Health ministry records reveal that an annual average of 310 deaths occurs each year. In other words, the mortality rate for Malins' Cliff is estimated at 31/100,000 (the same level as that for diphtheria outbreaks that used to occur during the last century).

Upon an initial investigation of the location, the health ministry identified two of the ten disaster incident locations where 80 percent of the deaths have occurred. In both of these locations, the international road is narrow and very close to the cliffside, where there are no guardrails. Six of the eight incidents have involved buses that fell over the cliffside to the road below. The situation is particularly challenging for NEMS because the accident often blocks either ingress or egress to this narrow canyon. This roadblock has resulted in delays of care that were directly attributable to poor health outcomes.

In partnership with the PIE program, the Pyronesia health ministry has established a system to use machine learning for automated monitoring and evaluation of the NEMS response. For this purpose, the health ministry developed a functional exercise involving patient transport to the hospital from the foot of Malins' Cliff. Field reports were automatically entered by sensor technology from the field into a remote, cloud-based management program provided by the PIE program. Rational agents were built for this system by specifying the event's task environment according to parameters that include the performance measure, environment, actuators, and sensors. In the case of emergency operations, the agent was a NEMS ambulance with the performance measure of the time elapsed between ambulance notification of emergency and hospital arrival with the patient. Sensors included synchronized clocks, commercial software for reporting traffic conditions, an accelerometer, and a global positioning system (GPS) located in each ambulance. Actuators included smartphones and the Internet for instant messaging intended to offer preventive or corrective actions. After one hour into exercise, statistically significant trends of increasing performance time (i.e., above three standard deviations) were found to be associated with a high probability of late hospital arrivals (i.e., performance defects). Unaware of highway traffic downstream, the local incident manager responded to this growing trend lighting up his dashboard by increasing resources (e.g., calling for more ambulances). However, performance times did not significantly change and instead increased and plateaued at an average time of six hours per patient. GPS tracking revealed that the same major bottleneck allowed for a rapid loading or patients but was followed by a five-hour traffic jam that occurred after the scene egress. Contrary to the incident manager's actions, the PIE system (with sensor inputs that also included traffic conditions and onboard accelerometers) began to notify other ambulances of the roadblock and divert them away using directions from commercially available traffic software.

Later, the data from the event was then analyzed for efficiency, effectiveness, and productivity. Most parameters were found to be unsatisfactory despite multiple practice drills and a full field exercise. The health ministry then turned to consider other hierarchical control measures for the reduction of these disaster-related deaths (see Figure 23.2). They recognized the need for additional plans beyond the mission area of response. This situation would require the creation of an emergency prevention plan. In doing so, the health ministry began to develop planning assumptions for the prevention of disaster-related deaths at Malins' Cliff.

First off, it was easily recognizable that the hazard could not be eliminated entirely. This international road was a lifeline for many citizens who did business and worked across the border. The mountainous region would also not allow for a suitable substitution. There were no alternate passes, and other means of transportation were cost-prohibitive. The health ministry did recommend implementing engineering controls – a local roadworks project that would install much-needed guardrails. In other words, a "fence," so to speak, at the top of the cliff that would prevent these frequent falls. The layered measure also involved administrative controls. The legislation was passed, requiring safety inspections for bus transport. Additional regulations were passed regarding driver training, licensure, and work hours, along with a lower speed limit for trucks and buses.

Finally, accelerometers were installed in all licensed buses with an automated variance alert system connected to the Pyronesia Bureau of Traffic Control.

Within one year, motor vehicle deaths dropped tenfold at Malins' Cliffs and 23 percent for the entire nation. These results were automatically imported into the PIE program knowledgebase and communicated to users through a monthly update. There, other users may interact with the same data to practice modeling their responses.

Appendix A: Epilogue

The Ambulance Down in the Valley

'Twas a dangerous cliff, as they freely
    confessed,
Though to walk near its crest was so
    pleasant;
But over its terrible edge there had slipped
A duke and full many a peasant.
So the people said something would have
    to be done,
But their projects did not at all tally;
Some said, "Put a fence 'round the edge
    of the cliff,"
Some, "An ambulance down in the valley."

But the cry for the ambulance carried
    the day,
For it spread through the neighboring city;
A fence may be useful or not, it is true,
But each heart became full of pity
For those who slipped over the dangerous
    cliff;
And the dwellers in highway and alley
Gave pounds and gave pence, not to put up
    a fence,
But an ambulance down in the valley.

"For the cliff is all right, if you're careful,"
    they said,
"And, if folks even slip and are dropping,
It isn't the slipping that hurts them so much
As the shock down below when they're
    stopping."
So day after day, as these mishaps occurred,
Quick forth would those rescuers sally
To pick up the victims who fell off the cliff,
With their ambulance down in the valley.

Then an old sage remarked: "It's a marvel
    to me
That people give far more attention
To repairing results than to stopping the
    cause,
When they'd much better aim at
    prevention.

Let us stop at its source all this mischief,"
    cried he,
"Come, neighbors and friends, let us rally;
If the cliff we will fence, we might almost
    dispense
With the ambulance down in the valley."

"Oh he's a fanatic," the others rejoined,
"Dispense with the ambulance? Never!
He'd dispense with all charities, too, if he
    could;
No! No! We'll support them forever.
Aren't we picking up folks just as fast as
    they fall?
And shall this man dictate to us? Shall he?
Why should people of sense stop to put up
    a fence,
While the ambulance works in the valley?"

But the sensible few, who are practical too,
Will not bear with such nonsense much longer;
They believe that prevention is better than
    cure,
And their party will soon be the stronger.
Encourage them then, with your purse,
    voice, and pen,
And while other philanthropists dally,
They will scorn all pretense, and put up
    a stout fence
On the cliff that hangs over the valley.

Better guide well the young than reclaim
    them when old,
For the voice of true wisdom is calling.
"To rescue the fallen is good, but 'tis best
To prevent other people from falling."
Better close up the source of temptation and
    crime
Than deliver from dungeon or galley;
Better put a strong fence 'round the top of
    the cliff
Than an ambulance down in the valley.

Joseph Malins (1895) [110]

Appendix B: Definition of Key Terms

Ability:	Possessing the means to accomplish a goal.
Absorptive capacity:	A limit to the rate or quantity of impact that can be absorbed (or assimilated to) to optimize outcome.
Accountability:	The acceptance of responsibility for performance and/or outcomes.
Accuracy:	The degree to which the result of a measurement conforms to the correct value or a standard. In other words, accuracy measures the validity of a measurement or test. Accuracy describes systemic errors and is measured as statistical bias.
Activation:	The action or process of making emergency operations active and the emergency plan operative.
Activity:	An action (or task) taken by an individual or group to achieve their aims.
Adaptive capacity:	A limit to the rate or quantity of incremental adjustments that may be made in the process to optimize outcome.
ADEPT™ planning wheel:	A design for planning that aligns preparedness goals with each of the five mission areas (i.e., phases) of emergency management (e.g., prevention, protection, mitigation, response, and recovery). The cycle includes five phases: risk assessment; emergency operations planning; gap analysis; preparedness planning; and monitoring and evaluation.
ADEPT™ risk assessment decision tree:	A decision support tool that models steps for performing a risk assessment.
Affective:	Related to emotions or feelings.
All-hazard approach:	The design and implementation of emergency management strategies for the full range of likely emergencies or disasters, including those caused by all (e.g., natural and technological) hazards.
Analysis:	The process of breaking a complex system into smaller parts in order to gain a better understanding of it.
Anecdotal:	Information that is based upon personal accounts rather than facts or research.
Application:	A computer program that performs a particular task or set of tasks.
Approach:	A perspective or method intended to improve the likelihood of success.
Artificial intelligence:	A branch of computer science dealing with the simulation of intelligent behavior in computers.

Assumption:	A fact or statement that is assumed to be true, when uncertainty exists.
Assumption-based planning:	A tool for identifying as many of the assumptions underlying the plans of an organization as possible and bringing those assumptions explicitly into the planning process.
B-tree:	A self-balancing tree data structure that is particularly well suited for storage systems that read and write relatively large blocks of data.
Basic plan:	The part of an emergency operations plan that provides an overview of the jurisdiction's emergency response organization and policies.
Bias:	Statistical description of the degree to which the expected value of the results differs from the true underlying quantitative parameter being estimated. Bias is the statistical representation of accuracy.
Black swan:	An unpredictable or unforeseen (i.e., low to no probability) event that results in a high impact but was not considered in previous risk assessments.
Bloom's taxonomy:	A classification system used to define and distinguish different levels of human cognition (e.g., thinking, learning, and understanding).
Capability:	The ability to achieve a desired operational effect under specified standards and conditions through combinations of means and ways to perform a set of tasks.
Capability-based planning:	Planning, under uncertainty, to provide capabilities suitable for a wide range of modern-day challenges and circumstances while working within an economic framework that necessitates choice.
Capability inventory:	A listing of available emergency-oriented resources during day-to-day and disaster operations, categorized by capability. Also known as a resource inventory that is compiled after resource typing.
Capacity:	The combination of all the strengths, attributes, and resources available within a community, society, or organization that can be used to achieve agreed goals.
Catastrophe:	A sudden and usually unforeseen disruption that exceeds the ability of the affected community to cope even using outside resources.
Certainty:	The absence of measurable error associated with estimation of an unknown value.
Channels of communication:	A functional pathway for communication among stakeholders.
Cognition:	Mental processes.

Cognitive:	Related conscious intellectual activity (e.g., thinking, reasoning, or remembering).
Common cause variation:	A fluctuation caused by unknown factors resulting in a steady but random distribution of output around the average of the data. Common cause variation is considered as a "natural" pattern, while special causes are unusual, not previously observed, non-quantifiable variation.
Common operational picture:	The single identical display of relevant (operational) information shared by more than one incident command system.
Community-based:	An activity that is organized and takes place locally.
Community engagement:	The process of working collaboratively with and through groups of people affiliated by geographic proximity, special interest, or similar situations to address issues affecting the well-being of those people.
Community preparedness:	The ability of communities to prepare for activities that will prevent, protect from, mitigate, respond to, and recover from the impact of disasters.
Community readiness:	A model for assessing how prepared the community is to take action to address a particular health issue.
Competency-based learning:	An approach to education that focuses on the student's demonstration of desired learning outcomes (i.e., competencies) as central to the learning process.
Competent:	Able to demonstrate the desired knowledge, skills, and behaviors necessary to successfully perform an activity.
Compliance:	Conforming to a rule, such as a specification, policy, standard or law.
Compliance management:	The process by which managers plan, staff, organize, control, and lead activities that ensure compliance with laws and standards.
Computing platform:	The digital environment in which a piece of software program code is executed (e.g., hardware, operating systems, web browsers or other underlying software).
Concept of operations:	A broad outline of assumptions regarding an operation or operations. The concept of operations is frequently embodied in operation plans, particularly when the plans cover a series of connected operations to be carried out simultaneously or in succession. Also called CONOPS.
Consensus:	A group decision-making process that not only seeks the agreement of most participants, but also to resolve or mitigate the objections of the minority to achieve the most agreeable decision.

Consequence:	The result or effect when a vulnerable asset is exposed to a disaster hazard.
Contingency:	A provision for an unforeseen event or circumstance.
Contingency plan:	A type of plan that describes alternate short-term activities for achieving objectives, when originally planned activities turn out to be impossible or ineffective.
Control theory:	A branch of mathematics and engineering, which defines the conditions needed for a system to maintain a controlled output in the face of input variation.
Controlling:	A management function that involves measuring and correcting processes to ensure that activities accomplish goals of a group.
Core capabilities:	Distinct abilities that are critical to accomplish strategic goals.
Core competency:	A modern management theory that relates the resources and capabilities that comprise the strategic advantage of an organization. As applied to education, core competencies are descriptions of the demonstrable knowledge, skills, and abilities to complete a strategic goal.
Core Planning Team (CPT):	A small group of individuals (led by a lead planner) given the primary responsibility of defining, creating, measuring, analyzing, improving, and controlling a plan.
Cost-benefit analysis:	A systematic approach to estimating the strengths and weaknesses of alternatives used to determine options which provide the best approach to achieving benefits while preserving resources.
Critical success factor:	A management term for an element that is necessary for an organization or project to achieve its mission.
Dashboard:	An information management tool that visually tracks, analyzes, and displays key performance indicators (KPI), metrics, and key data points to monitor a process or operation.
Data:	Facts and statistics compiled for reference or analysis.
Data component:	A basic unit of information having a meaning and that may have subcategories (data items) of distinct units and values. Also known as a data element or data point.
Data schema:	The organization of data described in a formal language supported by the database management system.
Data sharing:	The ability to share the same data resource with multiple applications or users.
Data structure:	A data organization, management, and storage format that enables efficient access and modification (e.g., tree data structures).

Database:	A structured or organized collection of data entities, which is accessed by a computer.
Database management system:	A computer application program that accesses or manipulates the database.
Decision tree:	A decision support tool that models decisions according to their probability, costs, and utility.
Defect:	A physical, functional, or esthetic attribute of a product or service that exhibits that the product or service failed to meet one of the desired specifications.
Delphi method:	A forecasting process framework based on the results of multiple rounds of questionnaires sent to a panel of experts.
Deming's cycle:	Also known as PDCA (plan–do–check–act), this is an iterative management method for the continuous improvement of processes and products that is based upon the scientific method of generating a hypothesis, testing it, and then evaluating the results before committing to an action.
Demobilization:	The process for a return of operations, facilities, and resources to routine, pre-incident status.
Disability:	Any condition of the body or mind (impairment) that makes it more difficult for the person with the condition to do certain activities (activity limitation) and interact with the world around them (participation restrictions).
Disaster:	A serious disruption of the functioning of a community or a society involving widespread human, material, economic, or environmental losses and impacts, which exceeds the ability of the affected community or society to cope using its own resources.
Disaster-related health risk:	An adverse event or negative health consequence caused by a disaster-related hazard.
Disaster risk:	The probability that a disaster will occur.
Disaster risk management:	The systematic process of using administrative directives, organizations, and operational skills and capacities to implement strategies, policies, and improved coping capacities in order to lessen the adverse impacts of hazards and the possibility of disaster.
Disaster risk reduction (DRR):	The concept and practice of reducing disaster risks through systematic efforts to analyze and manage the causal factors of disasters, including through reduced exposure to hazards, lessened vulnerability of people and property, wise management of land and the environment, and improved preparedness for adverse events.
Dose:	A measure of the quantity of exposure to a hazard.

Dose rate:	A measure of the rate of exposure to a hazard.
Dose–response modeling:	A modeling of the relationship between the magnitude of the response of an organism, as a function of exposure to a hazard after a certain exposure time (i.e., dose rate).
Early warning system (EWS):	Systems that generate and disseminate warning information to enable those threatened by a hazard to prepare and to act appropriately and in sufficient time to reduce the possibility of harm or loss.
Echelon:	An organizational structure in which subdivisions are placed one behind another, with a lateral and even spacing to the same side.
Effectiveness:	The degree to which objectives accomplish a desired outcome.
Efficacy:	A measure of the performance of an intervention under controlled circumstances.
Efficiency:	The ratio of the resources expended per activities accomplished by a process.
Egalitarian:	Relating to or believing in the principle that all people are equal and deserve equal rights and opportunities.
Emergency:	A sudden and usually unforeseen event that calls for immediate measures to minimize its adverse consequences.
Emergency management:	The managerial function charged with creating the framework within which communities reduce vulnerability to hazards and cope with disasters.
Emergency operations:	Activities performed during the response phase (i.e., mission area) of emergency management.
Emergency operations center (EOC):	A central facility where incident command and control activities are performed during the response phase (i.e., mission area) of emergency management.
Emergency operations plan (EOP):	A type of plan that describes activities performed during the response phase (i.e., mission area) of emergency management.
Emergency preparedness:	A program of long-term development activities whose goals are to manage all types of emergencies and bring about an orderly recovery.
Empirical:	Information that is based on verifiable observation or experience rather than theory or pure logic.
Empirical cycle:	The logical framework for a process of hypothesizing and then testing this hypothesis against verifiable observation or experience (rather than theory) in a systematic and rigorous approach.

End-user:	The person who uses a particular product or method.
Epidemiology:	The study of disease incidence, distribution, and control and other factors relating to health.
Essential elements of information:	Any critical intelligence information required by end-users to perform their mission.
Evacuation:	A population protection measure intended to remove occupants from hazardous areas during an emergency.
Evaluation:	The systematic determination of a project or program's merit, worth and significance, using criteria governed by a set of standards.
Evidence-based decision-making:	The practice of using scientific evidence to inform or guide decisions.
Exercise:	An instrument to train for, assess, practice, and improve performance in prevention, protection, response, and recovery capabilities in a risk-free environment.
Exposure:	People, property, systems, or other elements present in hazard zones that are thereby subject to potential losses.
Extensible Markup Language (XML):	A metalanguage which allows users to define their own customized markup (display) languages, especially in order to display documents on the internet.
Facilitator:	A neutral moderator that assists a group of people to work together better, understand their common objectives, and plan how to achieve these objectives, during meetings or discussions.
Feedback loop:	An engineering process in which the outputs of a system are circled back and used as inputs. Feedback is extensively used in control theory.
Function:	Any of a group of related actions contributing to a larger action (especially if it is specifically designed to accomplish the larger action).
Functional ability:	The actual or potential means to perform the activities that are expected.
Functional annex:	The part of the EOP that provides specific information and direction, typically focused on operations.
Gap analysis:	A process used to examine current performance with desired, expected, or target performance – often used to determine effectiveness and efficiency.
Goal:	The object of an effort. It is the aim or desired result of a work activity. In this book, the term "goal" is used interchangeably with "objective." The term "goal" is also here (arbitrarily) associated with strategy and the term "objective" is used with operations.

Governance:	The processes of interaction and decision-making among the actors involved in a collective problem that leads to the creation, reinforcement, or reproduction of social norms and institutions.
Group-based decision-making:	Also known as collaborative decision-making, a process by which individuals used evidence-based methods to collectively make a choice from the alternatives before them.
Group facilitation:	A process in which a person who is substantively neutral, and who has no substantive decision-making authority, diagnoses and intervenes to help a group improve how it identifies and solves problems and makes decisions, to increase the group's effectiveness.
Hazard:	A dangerous phenomenon, substance, human activity, or condition that may cause loss of life, injury, or other health impacts, property damage, loss of livelihoods and services, social and economic disruption, or environmental damage.
Hazard analysis:	The process of collecting and evaluating information on hazards and the conditions leading to their presence to determine which hazards are significant for health and should therefore be addressed in mission area planning.
Hazard characterization:	A description of the relationship between levels of a hazard exposure (dose) and the probability of subsequent development and severity of illness or other adverse health outcome (response).
Hazard identification:	The initial step of risk assessment in which the hazards are identified for further investigation.
Hazard-impact matrix:	Also known as a "hazard prioritization matrix," a visual representation of the risks presented as a graph, rating them by category of hazard probability (i.e., likelihood) and impact (i.e., severity of consequences).
Hazard map:	A map depicting the probability of a particular hazard occurrence within a specific location.
Hazard prioritization:	A component of risk analysis where risks are ranked according to their joint probability and impact.
Health hazard:	Chemical, physical, or biological factors in the environment that can have negative impacts on our short- or long-term health.
Health risk:	An adverse event or negative health consequence due to a specific event, disease, or condition.
Hierarchical format:	An organizational structure in which items are presented according to levels of importance.
Hierarchy of hypotheses:	The management approach (based up the "hierarchy of objectives") used to integrate strategic, operational, and tactical planning assumptions.

Hierarchy of plans:	The management approach (based up the "hierarchy of objectives") used to integrate strategic, operational, and tactical plans.
Hierarchy of process control:	The management approach (based up the "hierarchy of objectives") that applies a layered approach to integrate process control at various levels (e.g., elimination, substitution, engineering, administration, resource allocation).
Hierarchy tree:	A structure used to describe an approach to ranking, where items are sub-divided in a manner resembling branches on a tree.
Horizontal management:	A form or management with few or no levels of middle management between staff and executives. This usually involves peer-to-peer management.
Hotwash:	The immediate "after-action" discussions and evaluations of an agency's (or multiple agencies') performance following an exercise, training session, or major event.
Hyperlink:	A digital link from a hypertext file or document to another location or file, typically activated by clicking on a highlighted word or image on the screen.
Hypothesis:	A supposition or proposed explanation made on the basis of limited evidence as a starting point for further investigation.
Impact:	A measure of the severity of consequences caused by disaster hazards.
Impact analysis:	The component of risk assessment that involves quantifying the degree of damage or losses (e.g., disease) that may be expected when a vulnerable population is exposed to a hazard.
Incidence:	The occurrence, rate, or frequency of a disease, crime, or something else undesirable.
Incident:	An event or occurrence.
Incident action plan (IAP):	A type of plan that describe activities (short-term ways of achieving emergency response objectives) when original planning assumptions turn out to be wrong.
Incident command system (ICS):	An organizational system for managing emergency incidents that integrates response capabilities within a common organizational structure.
Incident manager:	The individual in charge of managing emergency response operations according to a structured incident command system.
Index:	A figure in a system or scale representing the average value of specific items as compared with some reference figure. It is a measurement constructed by summing up other, simpler, measurements.

Information:	A set of data that is processed in a meaningful way according to a given requirement.
Information exchange:	The bidirectional transmission or transfer of information, usually through electronic means.
Inputs:	That which is put in, taken in, or operated on by a process or system.
Integrated preparedness system:	A system that involves the coordinated management of preparedness programming for all five mission areas (i.e., phases) of emergency management (e.g., prevention, protection, mitigation, response, and recovery).
Intelligence:	The ability to apply knowledge to understand and predict future events through a series of procedures that refine data for prediction of future outcomes.
Job action sheets:	Job descriptions typically included in disaster plans that detail immediate, intermediate, and extended responsibilities of that position during emergency operations.
Judgment:	The ability to make decisions and draw conclusions.
Key performance indicator (KPI):	A quantifiable measure used to evaluate the success in meeting objectives for performance.
Knowledge:	Awareness gained by cognition (i.e., thought, experience, and the senses).
Knowledge, skills, and abilities (KSAs):	A description of qualifications related to the ability to successfully complete an activity.
Lead planner (LP):	A leader given the primary responsibility of managing a small group of individuals charged with defining, creating, measuring, analyzing, improving, and controlling a plan.
Leading:	A management function that involves influencing the manner in which people contribute to group goals.
Logical framework approach:	A management tool mainly used in the design, monitoring, and evaluation of humanitarian assistance and development projects.
Machine learning:	The subset of artificial intelligence that involves the study of computer algorithms which improve automatically through experience.
Majority rule:	The principle that the greater number should exercise greater power.
Management:	The process of designing and maintaining an environment (or system) in which individuals working together in groups efficiently accomplish selected aims.
Management by objectives (MBO):	A strategic management model where employees have a say in planning, as well as aligning objectives across the organization.

Mandate:	An official order or commission to do something.
Mass care:	The capability to provide congregated sheltering, feeding, emergency supplies, and reunification of families.
Mass casualty incident (MCI):	Any event that creates a number of casualties that exceed the resources normally available from local resources.
Measures of effectiveness:	Often expressed as probabilities, these measures are designed to correspond to accomplishment of mission objectives and achievement of desired outcome (i.e., objectives).
Measures of efficiency:	Often expressed as a rate, these measures relate the quality of performance in terms of resources used per outcome accomplished.
Measures of success:	A quantifiable expression of successful performance collected during the execution of a process (i.e., activities).
Memorandum of understanding (MOU):	A type of agreement that expresses a common understanding and intended common line of action, without legal commitment.
Microsoft Access™:	A commercially available database management system that combines a relational database engine with a graphical user interface and software-development tools.
Microsoft Excel™:	A commercially available spreadsheet that features calculation, graphing tools, pivot tables, and a macro programming language.
Microsoft SQL Server™:	A commercially available relational database management system which may run either on the same computer or on another computer across a network (including the Internet).
Microsoft Word™:	A commercially available word processor software.
Mitigation:	The lessening or limitation of the adverse impacts of hazards and related disasters.
Modeling:	Using a mathematical model that embodies a set of statistical assumptions concerning sample data (and similar data from a larger population.
Monitoring and evaluation:	A method used to assess the performance by continuous assessment and examination of activities according to objectives.
Morbidity:	Any departure from a state of physiological or psychological well-being. In practice, morbidity encompasses disease, injury, and disability.
Mortality:	The state of being subject to death.
Multi-sectoral approach:	An approach to emergency preparedness that involves input from the entire society (public and private) across all sectors.
Mutual aid agreement (MAA):	An agreement among emergency responders to lend assistance across jurisdictional boundaries.

Natural hazard:
Natural process or phenomenon that may cause loss of life, injury or other health impacts, property damage, loss of livelihoods and services, social and economic disruption, or environmental damage.

Negotiation:
A discussion aimed at reaching agreement.

Non-relational data:
Data that does not use the tabular schema of rows and columns found in most traditional database systems.

02C3 planning:
A planning model that combines five approaches for effective planning (i.e., operational-level, objective-based, capability-based, consensus-based, and compliant with population norms and regulations).

Objective:
The object of an effort. It is the aim or desired result of a work activity. In this book, the term "goal" is used interchangeably with objective.

Operational debriefing:
A review of the management of an emergency or critical incident to affirm and reinforce what worked well and refine and improve future processes and practice.

Operational intelligence:
Real time, or near real-time intelligence, often derived from technical means, and delivered immediately.

Operational objective:
Short-term aims or desired results whose achievement brings an organization closer to its long-term strategic goals.

Operational period:
The time scheduled for executing a given set of operation actions, as specified in a plan, usually according to work shift or day.

Operations:
A group of processes that are implemented by an organization according to a strategy.

Operations management:
A sub-discipline of management science concerned with designing and controlling the production of goods or services.

Operations plan:
A type of plan that describes the accomplishment of short-term objectives, in terms of activities.

Operations research:
The application of scientific methods to the study of alternatives in a problem situation.

Organizing:
A management function that involves establishing a system for coordinating activities to facilitate the goals of the group.

Outcome:
The intended goal or objective.

Output:
Actions or items that contribute to achieving an outcome (i.e., an intended goal or objective).

Pareto analysis:
A formal technique for selecting from multiple possible courses of action. The analysis is based on the idea that 80 percent of a project's benefit can be achieved by doing 20 percent of the work or conversely 80percent of problems are traced to 20 percent of the causes.

Partnership of equals:	Collaborations in which the participants each feel equally valued and equally respected.
Pathophysiologic:	A disordered physiological process associated with disease or injury.
Plan:	A design for achieving goals.
Planning:	The process of creating plans.
Planning assumptions:	An assertion about some characteristic of the uncertain future that, if negated, would lead to significant changes in the plan.
Planning Workgroup (PW):	A group of plan stakeholders representing multiple agencies, typically convened to create, execute, monitor, and evaluate a mission area plan.
Peer-to-peer network:	A distributed system or group of interconnected people that are equally privileged, equipotent participants in the application.
Performance:	The process of accomplishing an activity, process, or operation.
Performance indicators:	A type of performance measurement used to evaluate the successful accomplishment of a particular activity according to measurable standards.
Performance management:	The process of ensuring that a set of activities and outputs meets an organization's goals in an effective and efficient manner.
Performance measure:	An objective quantification of performance over time.
Points of contact:	An individual or group serving as the focal point of information concerning an activity or program when information is time sensitive and accuracy is important.
Population:	A particular selection, group, or type of people living in a specific area.
Position:	A group of duties and responsibilities which require the services of an employee on a part-time or full-time basis and are usually described in a job or position description.
Position descriptions:	The written description of the duties and responsibilities associated with a position or job.
Precision:	The degree to which repeated measurements (under unchanged conditions) show the same results. In other words, precision measures the reproducibility of a test when compared to itself. Precision describes random errors and is measured as statistical variability.
Prediction:	The ability to forecast the nature of a future event.
Preparedness:	The knowledge and capacity to effectively anticipate, respond to, and recover from the impacts of likely, imminent, or current hazard events or conditions.

Preparedness cycle: A model used to depict emergency preparedness as an iterative cycle.

Preparedness plan: A plan intended to guide a continuous cycle of planning, organizing, training, equipping, exercising, evaluating, and taking corrective action in an effort to ensure effective coordination during each phase (i.e., mission area) of the emergency management cycle (e.g., prevention, protection, mitigation, response, recovery).

Preparedness plan for response (PPR): A plan made to ensure a state readiness to prevent, protect from, mitigate the effects of, respond to, or recover from a disaster.

Prevalence: Sometimes referred to as prevalence rate, is the proportion of persons in a population who have a particular disease or attribute at a specified point in time or over a specified period of time.

Prevalent: Widespread in a particular area or at a particular time.

Prevention: The outright avoidance of adverse impacts of hazards and related disasters.

Preventive control: One of three types of control (i.e., detective, preventive, and corrective), these are internal controls put in place to avert a negative event from occurring.

Principle: A fundamental proposition that serves as the foundation for a chain of reasoning.

Probabilistic analysis: An approach to estimate the computational complexity of an algorithm or a computational problem.

Process: A set of activities (i.e., tasks) that are interrelated or that interact with one another.

Process control: The management function of active changing of the process based on the results of process monitoring.

Process control analysis: A statistical method to evaluate the control of a process.

Process management: The aligning of processes with an organization's strategic goals, designing and implementing process architectures, establishing process measurement systems that align with organizational goals, and educating and organizing managers so that they will manage processes effectively.

Processing: Subjecting something to a series of actions in order to achieve a particular result.

Productivity: A measure of the efficiency of a process, it is calculated by measuring the relative number of inputs required to produce outputs and/or outcomes.

Program: A set of related measures or activities with a particular long-term aim.

Program management:	A continuous process of managing several related projects, with the goal of improving performance.
Project:	A specific, finite activity that produces observable and measurable outcomes and/or outputs, under pre-determined requirements.
Project management:	A process of managing activities to achieve goals within a specified time.
Project management triangle:	Also known as the "iron triangle," this is a model of the constraints of project management contending that the quality of work is constrained by the project's budget, deadlines, and scope (features). The project manager can trade between constraints, but changes in one constraint necessitate changes in others to compensate or quality will suffer.
Prospective:	Relating to or effective in the future.
Protection:	Actions taken to deter threats, reduce vulnerabilities, and minimize the consequences associated with an incident.
Psychomotor:	Relating to the origination of movement in conscious mental activity. It is the relationship between cognitive functions and physical movement.
Qualitative description:	Descriptions or distinctions are based on some quality or characteristic rather than on some quantity or measured value.
Quality:	The totality of features and characteristics of a product or service that bear on its ability to satisfy given needs.
Quality control:	A business system of maintaining standards in products and/or services by testing a sample of the output against a standard specification or intended outcome.
Quantitative analysis:	A research method that focuses on quantifying the collection and analysis of measurable data. This can be compared to qualitative research that relies on data obtained by the researcher from first-hand observation, interviews, questionnaires, focus groups, participant-observation, recordings made in natural settings, documents, and artifacts.
Quantitative measure:	Information or data is based on quantities obtained using a quantifiable measurement process.
Recovery:	The restoration, and improvement where appropriate, of facilities, livelihoods, and living conditions of disaster-affected communities, including efforts to reduce disaster risk factors.
Relational data:	A type of data that is related to other data points.

Reliability:	The degree to which repeated measurements (under unchanged conditions) show the same results. In other words, precision measures the reproducibility of a test as compared to itself. Reliability describes the degree of random errors and is measured as statistical variability.
Repeatable:	The degree to which repeated measurements (under unchanged conditions) show the same results. Same as reproducible.
Reproducibility:	The degree to which repeated measurements (under unchanged conditions) show the same results.
Resilience:	The ability of a system, community, or society exposed to hazards to resist, absorb, accommodate to, and recover from the effects of a hazard in a timely and efficient manner, including through the preservation and restoration of its essential basic structures and functions.
Resource:	A stock or supply of assets (e.g., money, materials, and staff) that can be drawn upon in order to function effectively.
Resource allocation:	The assignment of available resources to various uses.
Resource management:	The efficient and effective development of an organization's resources when they are needed.
Response:	Activities that address the short-term, direct effects (consequences) of an incident. The provision of emergency services and public assistance during or immediately after a disaster to save lives, reduce health impacts, ensure public safety, and meet the basic subsistence needs of the people affected.
Response capacity:	The combination of all the strengths, attributes, and resources available within a community, society, or organization that can be used to achieve response goals in reaction to an emergency.
Responsible party:	A person or group of people that have an obligation to accomplish a particular activity.
Retrospective:	Pertaining to past events or situations.
Risk:	The probability of harmful consequences, or expected losses (deaths, injuries, property, livelihoods, economic activity disrupted, or environment damaged) resulting from interactions between natural or human-induced hazards and vulnerable conditions.
Risk assessment:	A methodology to determine the nature and extent of risk by analyzing potential hazards and evaluating existing conditions of vulnerability that together could potentially harm exposed people, property, services, livelihoods, and the environment on which they depend.

Risk characterization:	The estimation of the probability of occurrence and severity of potential adverse health effects, based on the preceding steps of hazard and impact analysis.
Risk equation:	A simplified mathematical formula used to represent the interaction between hazards and their impact, in terms of the probability of harmful consequences or losses.
Risk management:	An international standard (ISO 31000) for forecasting and evaluation of risks together with the identification of procedures to avoid or minimize their impact.
Run charts:	A graph that displays observed data in a time sequence. The data typically represents some aspect of the output or performance of a business process.
Satisfaction:	A customer-focused measure of quality regarding how well products and services supplied meet or surpass customer expectations.
Scale:	An index representing the ordinal ranking of the differences in intensity regarding one attribute of the same variable.
Scenario:	A postulated sequence or development of events, commonly used in planning.
Scenario-based planning:	Planning based upon assumptions made about a predicted future sequence of events.
Scientific method:	A procedure consisting of systematic observation, measurement, and experiment, and the formulation, testing, and modification of hypotheses.
Server:	A computer that provides data to other computers.
Shelter in place:	A population protection measure that directs people to stay in the indoor place or building that they already occupy and not to leave unless absolutely necessary.
Simulation:	A statistical and operational method using artificially generated data in order to test out a hypothesis or method.
Situation:	The location and set of circumstances surroundings a place or event.
Situation assessment:	A systematic process to gather, analyze, synthesize, and communicate data regarding environmental elements and events, time and space, the comprehension of their meaning, and the prediction of their future status.
Situational awareness:	The perception of environmental elements and events with respect to time or space, the comprehension of their meaning, and the projection of their future status.
Six Sigma™:	A quality control method used to improve the capability of their business processes by increasing performance and decreasing process variation. This leads to defect reduction and improvement in outcomes, employee morale, and quality of products or services.

Social vulnerability index (SVI) maps:	Census variables mapped at tract level to help local officials identify disaster-related health risk.
Software:	The entire set of programs, procedures, and routines associated with the operation of a computer system.
Staffing:	A management function that involves the alignment of worker knowledge, skills, and abilities to the appropriate process (i.e., set of activities) that will accomplish a group goal.
Stakeholder:	A person or organization with an interest or concern in something.
Standard:	A measurable norm for acceptability of quality.
Standard model:	A measurable norm for acceptable quality related to outcome.
Standardize:	To bring into conformity with a standard especially in order to assure consistency and regularity.
Standards of practice:	A measurable norm for acceptable quality related to performance.
Statistical power:	The likelihood that a statistical test will be able to detect an effect when one truly exists.
Statistical process analysis:	A statistical method to evaluate the control of a process.
Strategic capability:	The ability to accomplish long-term goals.
Strategic goal:	Long-term aims or desired results whose achievement brings an organization closer to its intended outcome.
Strategic plan:	A type of plan that describes the accomplishment of long-term goals, in terms of objectives.
Strategy:	A plan of action or policy designed to achieve a major overall aim.
Structured Query Language (SQL):	A computer programming language that is typically used in relational database or data stream management systems.
Surge capacity:	A measurable representation of the ability to manage a sudden influx of activity.
Susceptibility:	The state of being likely to be harmed by a particular hazard.
Sustainable development:	Development that meets the needs of the present without compromising the ability of future generations to meet their own needs.
Systems analysis:	The study of an activity to define its goals or purposes and to discover operations and procedures for accomplishing them most efficiently.
Systems theory:	The interdisciplinary study of systems.
Tactical plan:	A type of plan that describes short-term methods of managing resources to meet an objective.

Task: Also known as an activity, a piece of work to be undertaken or done.

Task analysis: The process of observing what steps it takes to perform a task for which there is a goal.

Technological hazard: A hazard originating from technological or industrial conditions, including accidents, dangerous procedures, infrastructure failures, or specific human activities that may cause loss of life, injury, illness, or other health impacts, property damage, loss of livelihoods and services, social and economic disruption, or environmental damage.

Threat: A dangerous phenomenon, substance, human activity or condition that is used to intentionally cause loss of life, injury or other health impacts, property damage, loss of livelihoods and services, social and economic disruption, or environmental damage.

Town hall meeting: Public meetings typically held between local and national officials to hear feedback from community members regarding topics of key interest.

Transformative capacity: A limit to the rate or ability to transform or change processes entirely to optimize outcome.

Unanimity: Agreement by all people involved.

Uncertainty: A state of limited knowledge where it is impossible to exactly describe the existing state, a future outcome, or more than one possible outcome. In statistics, it is the amount of measurable error associated with estimation of an unknown value.

Understanding: Perception of the significance, explanation, or cause of an event or occurrence.

Unified command: An organizational authority structure in which the role of incident commander is shared by two or more individuals, each already having authority in a different responding agency.

Usability: An international standard measure of intervention utility that is influenced by the effectiveness, efficiency, degree of satisfaction, and "freedom from risk" perceived among participants.

Validity: The degree to which the result of a measurement conforms to the true or correct value. In other words, validity measures the consistency of a test as compared to an external standard. Validity describes systemic errors and is measured as statistical bias.

Variability: A statistical value that measures the spread of a dataset around the mean.

Vertical management:	A form or management with respective levels of upper and middle management between staff and executives. Also known as top-down management.
Vulnerability:	The quality or state of being exposed to the possibility of being harmed. It is typically represented as the slope of the hazard dose–human response curve.
Work:	Any activity involving mental or physical effort done to achieve a purpose.

Appendix C: ADEPT Example Plan

Following is an example of ADEPT-style planning that uses Sphere Project international standards for humanitarian assistance as the content of the plan. (70) This example reveals how easily that standards for emergency response may be applied using the SOARR format.

In this example, Sphere planning guidance for water, supply, sanitation, and hygiene promotion (i.e., WASH) are described as the capability. The SOARR format is then used as a standard model for representing plan content. Plan stakeholders may then designate their own responsible parties and resources for each activity specified by the Sphere standards.

A more comprehensive ADEPT example plan (including the entire set of Sphere standards for humanitarian assistance) is available online at the following URL: https://spherestandards.org/handbook/.

This example plan includes the following Sphere standards:

- Common standards,
- WASH,
- Food security, nutrition, and food aid,
- Shelter settlement and non-food items, and
- Health services

Table A. Example of an ADEPT plan that organizes Sphere humanitarian standards into SOARR format

CAPABILITY	STRATEGIC GOAL	OPERATIONAL OBJECTIVE	ACTIVITY	RESPONSIBLE PARTY	RESOURCES
Sphere chapter title	Sphere section title in objective format	Sphere standard description	Sphere indicators	Position title	
Water Supply, Sanitation and Hygiene Promotion	Hygiene is promoted	All facilities and resources provided reflect the vulnerabilities, needs and preferences of the affected population. Users are involved in the management and maintenance of hygiene facilities where appropriate.	Identify the hygiene risks of public health importance.		Staffing Time Equipment Supplies Cost Essential elements of information
Water Supply, Sanitation and Hygiene Promotion	Hygiene is promoted	All facilities and resources provided reflect the vulnerabilities, needs and preferences of the affected population. Users are involved in the management and maintenance of hygiene facilities where appropriate.	Include an effective mechanism for representative and participatory input from all users, including in the initial design of facilities.		Staffing Time Equipment Supplies Cost Essential elements of information
Water Supply, Sanitation and Hygiene Promotion	Hygiene is promoted	All facilities and resources provided reflect the vulnerabilities, needs and preferences of the affected population. Users are involved in the management and maintenance of hygiene facilities where appropriate.	Provide equitable access to all the groups within the population, to the resources or facilities needed to continue or achieve the hygiene practices that are promoted.		Staffing Time Equipment Supplies Cost Essential elements of information

Table A. (cont.)

CAPABILITY	STRATEGIC GOAL	OPERATIONAL OBJECTIVE	ACTIVITY	RESPONSIBLE PARTY	RESOURCES
Sphere chapter title	Sphere section title in objective format	Sphere standard description	Sphere indicators	Position title	
Water Supply, Sanitation and Hygiene Promotion	Hygiene is promoted	All facilities and resources provided reflect the vulnerabilities, needs and preferences of the affected population. Users are involved in the management and maintenance of hygiene facilities where appropriate.	Address key behaviors and misconceptions in hygiene promotion messages and activities and target all user groups.		Staffing Time Equipment Supplies Cost Essential elements of information
Water Supply, Sanitation and Hygiene Promotion	Hygiene is promoted	All facilities and resources provided reflect the vulnerabilities, needs and preferences of the affected population. Users are involved in the management and maintenance of hygiene facilities where appropriate.	Include representatives from these groups in planning, training, implementation, monitoring and evaluation.		Staffing Time Equipment Supplies Cost Essential elements of information
Water Supply, Sanitation and Hygiene Promotion	Adequate water supply exists	All people have safe and equitable access to a sufficient quantity of water for drinking, cooking and personal and domestic hygiene. Public water points are sufficiently close to households to enable use of the minimum water requirement.	Provide water for drinking, cooking and personal hygiene in any household, at least 15 litres per person per day.		Staffing Time Equipment Supplies Cost Essential elements of information

Sector	Standard	Description	Key indicator	Planning elements
Water Supply, Sanitation and Hygiene Promotion	Adequate water supply exists	All people have safe and equitable access to a sufficient quantity of water for drinking, cooking and personal and domestic hygiene. Public water points are sufficiently close to households to enable use of the minimum water requirement.	The maximum distance from any household to the nearest water point is 500 metres.	Staffing · Time · Equipment · Supplies · Cost · Essential elements of information
Water Supply, Sanitation and Hygiene Promotion	Adequate water supply exists	All people have safe and equitable access to a sufficient quantity of water for drinking, cooking and personal and domestic hygiene. Public water points are sufficiently close to households to enable use of the minimum water requirement.	Queuing time at a water source is no more than 15 minutes (see guidance note 7).	Staffing · Time · Equipment · Supplies · Cost · Essential elements of information
Water Supply, Sanitation and Hygiene Promotion	Adequate water supply exists	All people have safe and equitable access to a sufficient quantity of water for drinking, cooking and personal and domestic hygiene. Public water points are sufficiently close to households to enable use of the minimum water requirement.	It takes no more than three minutes to fill a 20-litre container (see guidance notes 7–8).	Staffing · Time · Equipment · Supplies · Cost · Essential elements of information
Water Supply, Sanitation and Hygiene Promotion	Adequate water supply exists	All people have safe and equitable access to a sufficient quantity of water for drinking, cooking and personal and domestic hygiene. Public water points are sufficiently close to households to enable use of the minimum water requirement.	Maintain water sources and systems such that appropriate quantities of water are available consistently or on a regular basis.	Staffing · Time · Equipment · Supplies · Cost · Essential elements of information

Table A. (cont.)

CAPABILITY	STRATEGIC GOAL	OPERATIONAL OBJECTIVE	ACTIVITY	RESPONSIBLE PARTY	RESOURCES
Sphere chapter title	Sphere section title in objective format	Sphere standard description	Sphere indicators	Position title	
Water Supply, Sanitation and Hygiene Promotion	Adequate water supply exists	Water is palatable, and of sufficient quality to be drunk and used for personal and domestic hygiene without causing significant risk to health.	A sanitary survey indicates a low risk of faecal contamination.		Staffing Time Equipment Supplies Cost Essential elements of information
Water Supply, Sanitation and Hygiene Promotion	Adequate water supply exists	Water is palatable, and of sufficient quality to be drunk and used for personal and domestic hygiene without causing significant risk to health.	Ensure that there are no faecal coliforms per 100ml at the point of delivery.		Staffing Time Equipment Supplies Cost Essential elements of information

References

1. Federal Emergency Management Agency. *Developing and Maintaining Emergency Operations Plans, Comprehensive Preparedness Guide (CPG) 101, Version 2.0.* Washington, DC: Federal Emergency Management Agency; 2010.

2. Koontz H, Weihrich H. *Essentials of Management.* 5th ed. New York: McGraw-Hill; 1990.

3. Federal Emergency Management Agency. Guide for All-Hazard Emergency Operations Planning, State & Local Guide 101. 1996.

4. Federal Emergency Management Agency. *Incident Action Planning Guide.* Washington, DC: Department of Homeland Security; 2015.

5. Sobel M. *MBA in a Nutshell.* New York: McGraw-Hill; 2010.

6. Wren D. *The Evolution of Management Thought.* 3rd ed. New York: Wiley and Sons; 1987.

7. Federal Emergency Management Agency. *National Incident Management System.* Washington, DC: Department of Homeland Security; 2008.

8. Deming WE. *Out of the Crisis.* Cambridge, MA: Massachusetts Institute of Technology, Center for Advanced Engineering Study; 1986.

9. Tague NR. Plan–Do–Study–Act cycle. *The Quality Toolbox.* 2nd ed. Milwaukee, WI: American Society for Quality Press; 2005. p. 390–2.

10. Poister T, Aristigueta M, Hall J. *Managing and Measuring Performance in Public and Nonprofit Organizations.* San Francisco, CA: Jossey-Bass; 2015.

11. Hatry H. *Performance Measurement.* 2nd ed. Washington, DC: The Urban Institute Press; 2006.

12. Couillard J, Garon S, Riznic J. The Logical Framework Approach–Millennium. *Proj Manag J.* 2009;40(4):31–44.

13. Keim M. An innovative approach to capability-based emergency operations planning. *Disaster Health.* 2013;1(1):54–62.

14. Auf der Heide E. *Disaster Response: Principles of Preparation and Coordination.* St Louis, MO: Mosby; 1989.

15. United Nations International Strategy for Disaster Risk Reduction. UNISDR Terminology on Disaster Risk Reduction: United Nations International Strategy for Disaster Risk Reduction (UNISDR); 2009. Available from: www.unisdr.org/eng/library/UNISDR-terminology-2009-eng.pdf (last accessed May 27, 2021).

16. Duclos P, Sanderson L, Thompson FE, Brackin B, Binder S. Community evacuation following a chlorine release, Mississippi. *Disasters.* 1987;11(4):286–9.

17. Keim M. Environmental disasters. In: Frumkin H, ed. *Environmental Health from Global to Local.* 3rd ed. San Francisco, CA: John Wiley and Sons; 2016. p. 667–92.

18. Ciottone G. Introduction to disaster medicine. In: Ciottone G, ed. *Disaster Medicine.* Philadelphia, PA: Elsevier; 2016. p. 2–5.

19. Federal Emergency Management Agency. National Preparedness Goal: Department of Homeland Security; 2020. Available from: www.fema.gov/national-preparedness-goal (last accessed May 27, 2021).

20. Federal Emergency Management Agency. Mission Areas: Department of Homeland Security; 2020. Available from: www.fema.gov/mission-areas (last accessed May 27, 2021).

21. Keim M. Disaster preparedness. In: Ciottone G, ed. *Disaster Medicine.* 2nd ed. Philadelphia, PA: Mosby-Elsevier; 2016. p. 200–14.

22. Federal Emergency Management Agency. *Homeland Security Exercise and Evaluation Program (HSEEP).* Washington, DC: Department of Homeland Security; 2020.

23. Bazeyo W, Mayega RW, Orach GC, Kiguli J, Mamuya S, Tabu JS, Sena L, Rugigana E, Mapatano M, Lewy D, Mock N, Burnham G, Keim M, Killewo J. Regional approach to building operational level capacity for disaster planning: the case of the Eastern Africa region. *East Afr J Public Health*. 2013;10(2):447–58.

24. Keim M. History of the Pacific Emergency Health Initiative (PEHI). *Pac Health Dialog*. 2002;9(1):146–9.

25. Yi H, Zheng'an Y, Fan W, Xiang G, Chen D, Yongchao H, Xiaodong S, Hao P, Mahany M, Keim M. Public health preparedness for the world's largest mass gathering: 2010 World Exposition in Shanghai, China. *Prehosp Disaster Med*. 2012;27(6):589–94.

26. Sun X, Keim M, Dong C, Mahany M, Guo X. A dynamic process of health risk assessment for business continuity management during the World Exposition Shanghai, China, 2010. *J Bus Contin Emer Plan*. 2014;7(4):347–64.

27. Keim M, Runnels L, Lovallo A, Pagan Medina M, Roman Rosa E, Ramery Santos M, Mahany M, Cruz M. Measuring the efficacy of a pilot public health intervention for engaging communities of Puerto Rico to rapidly write hurricane protection plans. *Prehosp Disaster Med*. 2021;36(1):32–41.

28. Keim M. O2C3: A unified model for emergency operations planning. *Am J Disaster Med*. 2010;5(3):169–79.

29. de Boer J, Dubouloz M. *Handbook of Disaster Medicine*. The Netherlands: International Society of Disaster Medicine; 2000.

30. Lechat M. *Disaster as a Public Health Problem*. Belgium: Louvain University; 1985.

31. Federal Emergency Management Agency. *National Response Framework*. Washington, DC: Department of Homeland Security; 2008.

32. Henry R. *Defense Transformation and the 2005 Quadrennial Defense Review*. Washington, DC: Department of Defence; 2006.

33. Keim M, Giannone P. Disaster preparedness. In: Ciottone G, Darling R, Anderson P, Auf Der heide E, Jacoby I, Noji E, Suner S, eds. *Disaster Medicine*. 3rd ed. Philadelphia, PA: Mosby-Elsevier; 2006. p. 164–73.

34. Keim M. Defining disaster-related health risk: A primer for prevention. *Prehosp Disaster Med*. 2018;33(3):308–16.

35. Winderl T. *Disaster Resilience Measurements: Stock Taking of Ongoing Efforts in Developing Systems for Measuring Resilience*. New York: United Nations Development Program; 2014.

36. Dewar J, Builder C, Hix W, Levin M. *Assumption-Based Planning: A Planning Tool for Very Uncertain Times*. Santa Monica, CA: RAND Corporation; 1993.

37. Rumsfeld D. Defense Department Briefing Feb 12, 2002. Defense Department Briefing Feb 12, 2002: C-SPAN; 2002.

38. Sykes H, Dunham D. Critical assumption planning: A practical tool for managing business development risk. *J Bus Ventur*. 1995;10(6):413–24.

39. Provincial Emergency Program. *British Columbia Hazard Risk and Vulnerability Analysis Tool Kit*. Canada: Ministry of Public Safety and Solicitor General; 2004.

40. Standards Australia Committee OB-007. *AS/NZS 4360:2004 Risk Management. Sydney, Australia and Wellington*. New Zealand: Standards Australia International Ltd; 2004.

41. Doran G. There's a S.M.A.R.T. way to write management's goals and objectives. *Manag Rev*. 1981;70(11):35–6.

42. Drucker P. *The Practice of Management*. London: Butterworth-Heinemann; 2007.

43. Cobb J. Protagonist-driven urban ethnography. *City Community* 2015;14(4):4.

44. Wilson E. *Research Methods in Health Social Sciences*. Singapore: Springer; 2018.

45. Agerfalk P, Eriksson O. Socio-instrumental usability: IT is all about social action. *J Inf Tech*. 2006;21(1):24–39.

46. International Organization for Standardization. *Ergonomics of Human–System Interaction*. Geneva: IOS; 2018.

47. Lurie N, Manolio T, Patterson AP, Collins F, Frieden T. Research as a part of public

health emergency response *NEJM*. 2013;368(13):1251–5.

48. Institute of Medicine. *Enabling Rapid and Sustainable Public Health Research During Disasters: Summary of a Joint Workshop by the Institute of Medicine and the U.S. Department of Health and Human Services*. Washington, DC: National Academies Press; 2015.

49. Victora C, Bryce J. Evidence-based public health: Moving beyond randomized trials. *AJPH*. 2004;94(3):400–5.

50. Orach GC, Mamuya S, Mayega RW, Tabu SJ, Kiguli J, Keim M, Menya D, Mock N, Burnham G, Killewo J, Bazeyo W. Use of the Automated Disaster and Emergency Planning Tool in developing district level public health emergency operating procedures in three East African countries. *East Afr J Public Health*. 2013;10(2):439–46.

51. Sun X, Keim M, He Y, Mahany M, Yuan Z. Reducing the risk of public health emergencies for the world's largest mass gathering: 2010 World Exposition, Shanghai China. *Disaster Health*. 2013;1(1):21–9.

52. Swann J. How can we make better plans? *Higher Education Rev*. 1997;30(1):37–43.

53. Henry R. Transformation and the 2005 Quadrennial Defense Review. *Parameters*. 2005(Winter 2005–2006):5–15. Available from: www.comw.org/qdr/fulltext/05henry.pdf (last accessed May 27, 2021).

54. Bakken B. *Handbook on Long Term Defence Planning. Neuilly-Sur-Seine Cedex, France: Research and Technology Organization*. Contract No.: RTO technical report 69. 2003.

55. Davis P. *Analytic Architecture for Capabilities-Based Planning, Mission-System Analysis, and Transformation*. Santa Barbara, CA: RAND Corporation; 2002.

56. Federal Emergency Management Agency. *NIMS Components – Guidance and Tools*. Washington, DC: Department of Homeland Security; 2020. Available from www.fema.gov/emergency-managers/nims/components#icsr (last accessed May 27, 2021).

57. Dillard J, Schrader D. Reply: On the utility of the goals-plans-action sequence. *Commun Stud*. 1998;49(4):300–4.

58. Chim L, Nunez-Vaz R, Prandolini R. Capability-based planning for Australia's national security. *Security Challenges*. 2010;6(3):70–96.

59. TOGAF. *Capability-Based Planning*. Version 9.2. The Open Group; 2018 . Available from: https://pubs.opengroup.org/architecture/togaf9-doc/m/chap28.html#:~:text=Capability%2Dbased%20planning%20focuses%20on,to%20achieve%20the%20desired%20capability (last accessed May 27, 2021).

60. Medicine Io. In: *Committee on Guidance for Establishing Crisis Standards of Care for Use in Disaster S, editor. Crisis Standards of Care: A Systems Framework for Catastrophic Disaster Response*. Washington, DC: National Academies Press (US); 2012.

61. Murphy C, Gardoni P. The role of society in engineering risk analysis. A capabilities-based approach. *Risk Anal*. 2006;26(4):1073–83.

62. Murphy C, Gardoni P. Determining public policy and resource allocation priorities for mitigating natural hazards: A capabilities-based approach. *Sci Eng Ethics*. 2007;13:489–504.

63. Vroom V. Educating managers for decision-making and leadership. *Manag Decision*. 2003;41(10):968–78.

64. US Department of Homeland Security. *Planning Considerations: Evacuation and Shelter-in-Place Guidance for State, Local, Tribal, and Territorial Partners*. Washington, DC: US Department of Homeland Security; 2019.

65. The Sphere Project. *The Sphere Handbook*. 4th ed. Geneva: Practical Action Publishing; 2018.

66. Baccino-Astrada A. *Manual on the Rights and Duties of Medical Personnel in Armed Conflicts*. 2nd ed. Geneva: International Committee of the Red Cross and the League of Red Cross and Red Crescent Societies; 1982.

67. Heger T, Jeschke JM. The hierarchy-of-hypotheses approach updated – A toolbox for structuring and analysing theory, research and evidence. In Jeschke JM, Heger T, eds. *Invasion Biology: Hypotheses and Evidence*. Berlin: CABI, International; 2018. p. 38–48.

68. Leonard-Barton D. Core capabilities and core rigidities. *Strategic Manag J*. 1992;13 (Special issue):11–125.

69. International Organization for Standardization. ISO 31000 – Risk management a practical guide for subject matter experts: International Organization for Standardization; 2009. Available from: www.iso.org/standard/43170.html (last accessed May 27, 2021).

70. CDC. CfDC. *Lesson 3: Measures of Risk*. Atlanta, GA: Centers for Disease Control (CDC); 2012. Available from: www.cdc.gov/csels/dsepd/ss1978/lesson3/section2.html (last accessed May 27, 2021).

71. Wharton F. Risk management basic concepts in general principles. In: Ansell J, Wharton F, eds. *Risk Analysis Assessment and Management*. Chichester: John, Wiley & Sons; 1992. p. 100.

72. Association of Faculties of Medicine of Canada. *AFMC Primer on Population Health*. Ottawa: Association of Faculties of Medicine of Canada; 2017. Available from: http://phprimer.afmc.ca/Glossary?l=H (last accessed May 27, 2021).

73. Assistant Secretary for Preparedness and Response Technical Resources, Assistance Center, and Information Exchange. *Topic Collection: Hazard Vulnerability/Risk Assessment*. Washington, DC: US Department of Health and Human Services; 2017. Available from: https://asprtracie.hhs.gov/technical-resources/3/Hazard-Vulnerability-Risk-Assessment/0 (last accessed May 27, 2021).

74. United Nations International Strategy for Disaster Risk Reduction. *Terminology on Disaster Risk Reduction*. Geneva: United Nations International Strategy for Disaster Reduction; 2009. Available from: www.unisdr.org/files/7817_UNISDRTerminologyEnglish.pdf (last accessed May 27, 2021).

75. World Health Organization. *Glossary of Health Emergency and Disaster Risk Management Terminology*. Geneva: World Health Organization; 2020.

76. Centers for Disease Control and Prevention. Morbidity surveillance following the midwest flood – Missouri, 1993. *JAMA*. 1993;270(18):2164.

77. Keim M. Assessing disaster-related health risk: Appraisal for prevention. *Prehosp Disaster Med*. 2018;33(3):317–25.

78. Keim M. Developing a public health emergency operations plan: A primer. *Pac Health Dialog*. 2002;9(1):124–9.

79. Keim M. Disaster risk management for health. In Suresh S. David, ed. *Textbook of Emergency Medicine*. Chicago, IL: Wolters Kluwer Health (Lippincott); 2010. p. 1309–18.

80. Federal Emergency Management Agency. *The National Risk Index*. Washington, DC: Department of Homeland Security; 2020. Available from: https://hazards.geoplatform.gov/portal/apps/MapSeries/index.html?appid=ddf915a24fb24dc8863eed96bc3345f8 (last accessed May 27, 2021).

81. United Nations. *PreventionWeb*. Geneva: United Nations Office for Disaster Risk Reduction; 2020. Available from: www.preventionweb.net/english/ (last accessed May 27, 2021).

82. World Health Organization, Food and Agriculture Organization of the United Nations. *Hazard Characterization for Pathogens in Food and Water – Guidelines*. Geneva: World Health Organization and Food and Agriculture Organization of the United Nations; 2003.

83. Frost WH. Some conceptions of epidemics in general. *Am J Epidemiol*. 1976;103(2):141–51.

84. Keim M, Lee V, Cruz M, Reddick R, Heitgerd J, Kaplan B, Gregory E, Smith M, Manangan A, Calame P, Young R, Bullard S, Flanagan B, Liske K, Neurath B, Burger E. *The CDC/ATSDR Public Health Vulnerability Mapping System*. Atlanta, GA: Centers for Disease Control; 2007. Available from: https://ininet.org/the-

cdcatsdr-public-health-vulnerability-mapping-system-using.html (last accessed May 28, 2021).

85. Geospatial Research Analysis and Services Program. *The Social Vulnerability Index*. Atlanta, GA: Centers for Disease Control and Prevention; 2017. Available from: https://svi.cdc.gov/.

86. Badia A, Pallares-Barbera M, Valldeperas N, Gisbert M. Wildfires in the wildland–urban interface in Catalonia: Vulnerability analysis based on land use and land cover change. *Sci Total Environ*. 2019;673:184–96.

87. Endsley MR. Toward a theory of situation awareness in dynamic systems. *Human Factors*. 1995;37(1):32–64.

88. Anonymous. *Guide to Strategic Planning Process*. Washington, DC: Office of the Under Secretary of Defense for Acquisition & Sustainment; 2012. p. 1–10. Available from: www.acq.osd.mil/dpap/ccap/cc/jcchb/Files/Topical/AP_files/guides/Guide_to_Strategic_Planning_Process_2012.pdf (last accessed May 27, 2021).

89. Department of Homeland Security. *National Information Exchange Model (NIEM)*. Washington, DC: Department of Homeland Security; 2020. Available from: www.niem.gov/ (last accessed May 27, 2021).

90. Rosello V. *The Origins of Operational Intelligence*. School of Military Studies. Fort Leavenworth, KS: US Army Command and General Staff College; 1989. p. 1–54. Available from: https://apps.dtic.mil/sti/pdfs/ADA215754.pdf (last accessed May 27, 2021).

91. Negash S. Business intelligence. *Commun Assoc Inf Systems*. 2004;13:177–95.

92. James L. *Fail vs Finished: The Difference Between Information and Intelligence*. Southborough, MA: MIS Training Institute; 2017. Available from: https://misti.com/infosec-insider/fail-vs-finished-the-difference-between-information-and-intelligence (last accessed May 27, 2021).

93. Department of Homeland Security. *Information Sharing*. Washington, DC: Department of Homeland Security; 2020.

Available from: www.dhs.gov/information-sharing (last accessed May 27, 2021).

94. Keim ME, Noji E. Emergent use of social media: a new age of opportunity for disaster resilience. *Am J Disaster Med*. 2011;6(1):47–54.

95. US Department of Defense. *Dictionary of Military and Associated Terms, Joint Publication 1-02*. Washington, DC: US Department of Defense; 2008. p. 1–780.

96. Goldacre B, Harrison S, Mahtani K, Heneghan C. *Background Briefing for WHO consultation on Data and Results Sharing During Public Health Emergencies*. Oxford: World Health Organization (WHO), Sciences NDoPCH; 2015.

97. Bjerge B, Clark N, Fisker P, Raju E. Technology and information sharing in disaster relief. *PLoS One*. 2016;11(9):1–20.

98. Harvard Humanitarian Initiative. *Disaster Relief 2.0: The Future of Information Sharing in Humanitarian Emergencies*. Washington, DC: UN Foundation & Vodafone Foundation Technology Partnership; 2011.

99. Pyzdek T, Keller PA. *The Six Sigma Handbook*. 3rd ed. New York: McGraw-Hill; 2009. p. 47–67.

100. McCormick V. *NIOSH and the Hierarchy of Controls: Network Enviornmental Systems*; 2019. Available from: www.nesglobal.net/nioshs-hierarchy-of-controls/ (last accessed May 27, 2021).

101. Centers for Disease Control and Prevention. *Public Health Emergency Preparedness and Response Capabilities: National Standards for State, Local, Tribal, and Territorial Public Health*. Atlanta, GA: Centers for Disease Control and Prevention; 2020. Available from: www.cdc.gov/cpr/readiness/capabilities.htm (last accessed May 27, 2021).

102. Edwards R, Jumper-Thurman P, Plested B, Oetting E, Swanson L. Community readiness: Research to practice. *J Community Psychology*. 2000;28(3):291–307.

103. The Sphere Project. *Humanitarian Charter and Minimum Standards in Disaster Response*. Geneva: The Sphere Project; 2008.

104. Bolman L, Deal, T. *Reframing Organizations.* 2nd ed. San Francisco, CA: Jossey-Bass; 1997.

105. Chandler T. Use of reframing as a classroom strategy. *Education.* 1998;119 (2):365.

106. Berners-Lee T, Fischetti M. *Weaving the Web.* San Francisco, CA: Harper; 1999. p. 308–64.

107. DeSalvo KB, Wang YC, Harris A, Auerbach J, Koo D, O'Carroll P. Public Health 3.0: A call to action for public health to meet the challenges of the 21st century. *Prev Chronic Dis.* 2017;14:170017.

108. Gallaugher J. *Information Systems: A Manager's Guide to Harnessing Technology.* 1.4 ed. Irvington, NY: Flat World Knowledge, Inc.; 2012.

109. Russell S, Norvig P. *Artifical Intelligence: A Modern Approach.* Hoboken, NJ: Pearson Education; 2020.

110. Malins J. The Fence of the Ambulance. *Walton County Prevention Coalition.* Available from: https://static1.squarespace .com/static/55bfbea7e4b0c49b1b23b399/t/ 55ce42f2e4b06cc6fac64efb/1439580914646/ 15+PHM+Winter+2011-2012+The+Fence +or+the+Ambulance.pdf (last accessed May 27, 2021).

Index